Oxford Medical Publications

Presenting medical statistics from proposal to publication

Presenting Medical Statistics

From Proposal to Publication:
A Step-by-Step Guide

Janet L. Peacock
Professor of Health Statistics,
Brunel University, West London UK

and

Sally M. Kerry
Senior Lecturer in Medical Statistics,
St George's University of London UK

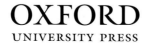

OXFORD

UNIVERSITY PRESS

Great Clarendon Street, Oxford OX2 6DP

Oxford University Press is a department of the University of Oxford.
It furthers the University's objective of excellence in research, scholarship,
and education by publishing worldwide in

Oxford New York

Auckland Cape Town Dar es Salaam Hong Kong Karachi
Kuala Lumpur Madrid Melbourne Mexico City Nairobi
New Delhi Shanghai Taipei Toronto

With offices in

Argentina Austria Brazil Chile Czech Republic France Greece
Guatemala Hungary Italy Japan Poland Portugal Singapore
South Korea Switzerland Thailand Turkey Ukraine Vietnam

Oxford is a registered trade mark of Oxford University Press
in the UK and in certain other countries

Published in the United States
by Oxford University Press Inc., New York

British Library Cataloguing in Publication Data

Data available

Library of Congress Cataloging in Publication Data

Peacock, Janet (Janet L.)
    Presenting medical statistics from proposal to publication: a step-by-step
guide/Janet L. Peacock and Sally M. Kerry.
        p. ; cm.
Includes bibliographical references and index.
  1. Medical statistics.   I. Kerry, Sally M.   II. Title.
[DNLM: 1. Statistics. 2. Publishing. WA 950 P356p 2006]
RA407.P43 2006
610.21—dc22   2006008850

Typeset by Newgen Imaging Systems (P) Ltd., Chennai, India
Printed in Great Britain
on acid-free paper by
Ashford Colour Press Ltd., Gosport, Hampshire

ISBN 0–19–859966–8 (Pbk.: alk.paper)   978–0–19–859966–1 (Pbk.)

10 9 8 7 6 5 4 3 2 1

Preface

The inspiration for this book has come from many years of designing, analysing and reporting medical research studies ourselves, and giving advice to medical practitioners, researchers and students. We have had a growing realisation that presenting statistics is rarely straightforward. While there are many good medical statistics textbooks, these do not cover in detail the practical issues which many researchers grapple with at various stages of the research process, of how to present statistics. We have therefore tried to set in print the principles and ideas that we have assimilated over the years and which we have advised others to use too.

During our careers in medical research we have been privileged to work with many different colleagues and the majority of examples in our book come from this rich source. We wish to thank our colleagues with whom we have collaborated in these research studies: Ross Anderson, Martin Bland, Maggie Bruce, Sandy Calvert, Franco Cappuccio, Iain Carey, Clare Chazot, Françoise Cluzeau, Derek Cook, Lyndsey Emmett, Anne Greenough, Phillip Hay, Sean Hilton, Alice Johnson, Samantha Johnson, Liz Limb, Neil Marlow, Louise Marston, Lesley Meyer, Pippa Oakeshott, Phil Peacock, Ruth Ruggles, Malcolm Stewart, Jane Scarlett, Andrew Steptoe, Glenn Stewart, David Strachan, Mark Thomas, Christina Victor. We also wish to thank the many researchers and students who over the years have come to see us for statistical advice, and also those whose grant proposals and submitted papers we have reviewed. We have learnt so much through you, even though you never knew it!

We wish to express special thanks to Martin Bland who has been an inspiration and encourager to us for many years and who has taught us so much about medical statistics. We are grateful to Martin and to Louise Marston for reading an earlier draft of our book and for making many helpful comments, although any errors or mistakes remain our own. We thank Phil Peacock for help in assembling the references. We are grateful for the support and patience shown us by the staff at Oxford University Press, especially when we were slow to deliver the manuscript. Finally, we wish to thank our longsuffering families, Eric, Jo, Rachelle, and Phil Peacock, and Graham, Paul, Philip, Sarah, and Sheila Kerry for their support throughout, and forbearance when we were at certain times constantly 'working on the book'.

JP & SK

Foreword

Evidence-based practice is now applied in all fields of healthcare: in medicine, nursing, physiotherapy, and even complementary therapy. It is advocated at every level, from individual patient care to health policy. Statisticians are usually very sympathetic to this view. For many, their original discipline was mathematics, which is entirely evidence-based; we do not know something until we can prove it, otherwise it is merely a hypothesis or conjecture. Statistics itself is the science of gathering, analysing, and interpreting numerical evidence, so naturally statisticians are strongly biased in evidence's favour. However, the entirely admirable notion of evidence-based practice came from within healthcare; it was not imposed from outside by statisticians or by any other group. As a result of developments in their own disciplines, healthcare professionals need to be able to read and use research evidence more than ever before. Statisticians are enthusiastic partners to help them to do it.

Evidence-based practice requires evidence, and more and more healthcare professionals find themselves faced with the need to collect and present research evidence themselves. The raw material of clinical research is usually patients, and access to patients and delivery of treatments to be evaluated are both via clinicians, whose primary concern is, quite rightly, their clinical practice. Clinical research is unusual in this, as in many fields most research is done by professional researchers. As a result, it has always been the case that many health researchers were inexperienced and carried out research in the time which they could spare from clinical practice. There are advantages to the wide involvement of clinicians in research, as some understanding of research is widespread among healthcare professionals and research evidence is something of which they can claim some ownership. The disadvantage is that for many research is a spare-time activity, and the actors are learning the basics as they go along.

The quality of health research has improved greatly during my time as a medical statistician. One feature of this improvement is a much greater emphasis on the importance of both good research design and good statistical analysis. At the same time, the availability of computers with powerful statistical programs such as SPSS and Stata has greatly extended the range of statistical techniques available to the researcher. What was once very difficult and rarely seen is now commonplace and researchers are expected to use quite complex statistical methods where appropriate.

In parallel with these developments, there is a requirement for healthcare workers to become more highly educated. Non-graduate professions are becoming graduate entry and post-graduate qualifications are becoming a requirement for professional development. Many healthcare professionals find themselves writing dissertations and theses. In the nature of dissertations, collaboration is not available and, although authors may get some statistical advice, they are very much on their own.

Health research is complicated, involves many different skills, and most research involves people from several disciplines. Multi-authored papers are common. If we are really lucky, one of these authors might be a statistician, but statisticians are rare birds and there are not enough for more than a small minority of projects to have a statistical collaborator. Even statistical advice can be hard to find.

There are many books, both good and bad, which will guide the researcher in the choice and interpretation of statistical analyses. There are books which describe how to use statistical software to carry out analyses. For the inexperienced researcher, the greatest problem is often taking the results of analyses performed using computer programs and turning these into a report, a paper for publication, or a dissertation or thesis. Janet Peacock and Sally Kerry are experienced advisers of researchers and teachers of students writing dissertations, and they saw a need for a book which concentrates on how to use these analyses to produce statistics to present.

The authors of this book and I go back a long way. I have written both research and educational papers with each of them, and a book with Janet Peacock. (We have never published anything by all three of us, until they asked me to write this foreword!) We have taught thousands of students together, both undergraduate and postgraduate, from a wide range of healthcare disciplines. Together Janet and Sally go back even further, to their student days. They work well together and I think that now they have produced a book which meets a real need for healthcare researchers working at every level from undergraduate project to multinational randomised controlled trial. I hope that you will be as happy with it as I am.

Martin Bland,
Professor of Health Statistics,
University of York, December 2005.

Contents

Dedicated to our families

Eric, Jo, Rachelle, Phil

Graham, Paul, Philip, Sarah, Sheila

CHAPTER 1

Introduction

1.1 The use of statistics in research

Medical statistics is the tool by which numerical information can be translated into evidence. This evidence might be for the cause of a disease or for the effectiveness of an intervention. The advent of evidence-based medicine has led to a greater demand for such research evidence.

The majority of researchers in medicine and the health care professions now use statistics in their research. It is easier than ever before for researchers to do their own statistical analyses using one of the many statistical programs available with their user-friendly interfaces. This is probably a mixed blessing.

On the positive side, researchers can now be independent and no longer have to rely on finding a friendly statistician to do analyses for them. The downside is that because statistical programs are easy to use, it is equally easy to do the wrong analysis. Even if the right analysis is performed, the programs often produce a large amount of output which tends to contain some relevant and some irrelevant results. Selecting the appropriate results from such output is not always straightforward. In addition, statistical programs, though very sophist-icated, do not generally tell the user whether a particular analysis is valid or not.

1.2 Presenting medical statistics

Research is conducted as part of a search for more knowledge. For the most part, the researcher fully intends to share newly gained knowledge with others so that they can benefit from the findings in future research, in professional practice, or in both. However, the sharing of research findings sometimes causes some difficulty. The presentation of statistical information is not straightforward, and yet inadequate presentation will fail to communicate the relevant information, and may even communicate misleading or incorrect information.

The CONSORT group, established in the 1990s, recognised this and has developed guidelines for the reporting of randomised trials. The group argues persuasively that to comprehend the results of a randomised trial, the reader must be able to understand all of the constituent parts of the study process, and that full and transparent presentation is needed to achieve this (Moher *et al.* 2001). It is clear that good presentation skills are crucial to all areas of evidence-based practice, so that other practitioners can critically assimilate and interpret evidence, and turn evidence into better practice.

1.3 This book

This book describes the presentation of required statistical information through the entire research process, from the development of the research proposal, through to applying for ethical approval, to analysing the data, and then writing up the results. We use the term 'statistical information' to include describing the study design, the calculation of sample size, and data processing, as well as the data analysis and reporting of results. It is written for researchers in medicine and in the professions allied to medicine.

The first part of the book describes the research process and discusses how to write a research protocol, and how to report the statistical aspects in ethical approval applications. We give general guidelines on writing up a study for different media such as a journal paper, a report, a dissertation or thesis, or an oral or poster presentation. The second part of the book illustrates how to present different analyses, going from simple descriptive analyses to more complex analyses such as survival analysis. Throughout the book we use examples and analyses from real research, mostly our own.

We give many examples of how to present statistical information for a proposal, a paper, or a report. We have usually used a concise format so that it is appropriate for a shorter report or journal paper but can easily be expanded to suit a longer document such as a dissertation or thesis. We show how the methods and results sections can be written and also give some discussion points to show how the interpretation of statistical findings might feed into the discussion section.

1.3.1 Statistical analyses and software

We use various statistical programs, commercial and free. The main analyses are performed in both Stata and SPSS. In addition, some sample size calculations are done in Epi-Info, and we use some free programs available on the web and written by friends and colleagues. We show how the results from statistical programs can be translated into text or tables for inclusion in a written document. We indicate which particular results in an output are relevant, and then give an example of how it can be presented and described.

We used Stata v8, although Stata v9, which had just arrived as we finished this book, has the same commands and will give the same output and answers. We used SPSS v12.0.

Where a study that we used has been published, we have given the reference so that readers can look at it if they wish. Sometimes we have simplified or reduced the original analyses where, for example, many variables had been included but only a few are needed to illustrate the point we wished to make.

1.3.2 References

The reference section at the end of the book includes books, journal articles, and websites. We have listed websites separately. In the text, websites are referenced using a shortened form (e.g. www.cdc.gov) and in the reference list we give the full address http://www.cdc.gov/epiinfo/.

1.3.3 Using this book

In our book we have given detailed descriptions as well as summary boxes to help readers who require different levels of detail. The boxes contain various types of material for quick access—helpful tips, examples, summaries, and information. In addition, each chapter contains a summary box with the main points covered in the chapter. The figures contain computer output with the commands needed to obtain them, markers to indicate key results which should be reported, and comments and notes.

Some readers will read straight through the book, and some will use it as a practical reference book to 'dip in and out', as needed.

Our book is not a textbook of medical statistics, but rather is a practical reference book. There are many good examples of medical statistics textbooks and we have cited some of these for reference. Some of our 'information' boxes give the theoretical and practical issues that need to be considered when reporting statistics, and we give references for further reading throughout the book.

Our references are not exhaustive. The books that we have cited are ones that we have on our bookshelves and with which we are are familiar. There are undoubtedly many excellent statistics books that we have not been able to mention; we apologise for this. The software that we have used is only a sample of all that is available. Researchers who use programs other than those used in this book will still find much useful information in the book.

We have used varying formats for presenting graphs, tables, and results in different parts of this book, to reflect the real world. Often, there is no single 'right' way to present findings, but there are often unhelpful or wrong ways of presentation. In this book we have made practical suggestions for presenting statistical information.

The chapters of the book frequently refer to other sections for other examples or more explanation, if required. However, each chapter is relatively self-contained, and therefore there is some repetition or reinforcement of material.

We have included the main steps in setting up a research study, and also have included all the analyses that we commonly use, as well as some more complex ones. There are certain to be analyses that we have not included. Also, as software and fashions change, different analyses become more widespread. The principles that we have given in this book will guide researchers in presenting statistical material in all parts of the research process with different study designs and different analyses.

1.3.4 Conventions used in the book

In the computer outputs, we have used *italics* for variable names and Stata commands are in **bold print**. SPSS has menus, and so we have indicated the command sequence in the relevant figure.

1.4 Final word

We have done our best to check all of our analyses and the presentations, but it is always possible that errors have slipped through. If you find any errors or mistakes in our book, please tell us and we will post corrections on the web (www.brunel.ac.uk).

CHAPTER 2

Introduction to the research process

2.1 Defining the research question

Often research begins with a general question in the researcher's mind such as 'I wonder why . . . ?' or 'I wonder if . . . ?', perhaps arising from an observation, as illustrated in Box 2.1. Such enquiry is an essential prerequisite to the research process but is not sufficient to design a study.

BOX 2.1 EXAMPLE

An observation

It was observed that several patients receiving treatment for hypertension reported improvement in migraine while taking lisinopril. This led to a randomised trial to address the following research questions (Schrader et al. *2001).*

- *Does lisinopril reduce the number of days affected by migraine, numbers of hours with headache, and number of days with headache?*

- *What is the reduction in blood pressure when lisinopril is prescribed to patients with normal blood pressure?*

A research study needs to have a specific question which the researcher wishes to answer. This might take the form of a simple question such as 'What is the prevalence of asthma in the UK?' Alternatively the research question may be a hypothesis to test such as 'Is the prevalence of asthma increasing?' In a study testing a hypothesis the researcher is looking for evidence for or against this hypothesis so that he can make an informed decision as to whether or not it is likely to be true.

However, even these questions are not sufficiently defined. The first example appears straightforward until we consider what is meant by 'asthma'? What age groups are we interested in? We then might tighten up our question to 'What is the prevalence of doctor-diagnosed asthma in adults in the UK?' Similar issues arise in the second example. We need to know what is meant by an increase? Over what time period? Thus we might refine our question to ask 'Has the prevalence of doctor-diagnosed asthma in adults increased in the past 10 years?' Other examples are shown in Box 2.2.

BOX 2.2 EXAMPLE

Examples of specific research questions

◆ *What is the prevalence of doctor-diagnosed asthma in adults in the UK?*

◆ *Has the prevalence of doctor-diagnosed asthma in adults increased in the past 10 years?*

◆ *What is the prevalence of chlamydia infection among asymptomatic women attending for cervical smear tests in inner city General Practices in the UK?*

◆ *Is miscarriage at less than 16 weeks associated with bacterial vaginosis infection diagnosed before 10 weeks gestation?*

These examples illustrate the importance of tightly defining our research question. Once we have a research question, then the required study design is easier to decide upon. In addition, the research question needs to be one that can be answered. For example, a published study sought to determine whether an episode of the TV programme *Casualty*, which involved a suicide, caused an increase in suicide rates in the population (Hawton *et al.* 1999). The researchers reported that an increase in the suicide rate was observed, but they concluded that they could not say if the episode actually caused the increase. That question is not answerable.

2.2 Writing a research protocol

A research protocol is a formal document outlining the proposed study. It is an essential part of the study design and conduct. It starts with the research question, discusses what is already known about the topic, and explains how the proposed study will further knowledge. The protocol describes the study design and provides details of how the study will be conducted, including a plan for any statistical analysis.

There are few occasions that we can think of in medical research where a protocol is unnecessary, and so we recommend that researchers always write one. The length and extent of detail required will vary; for example, a protocol for a small student project will be shorter than one needed for a multi-centre clinical trial where detailed instructions for conducting the study are essential to maintain uniformity. We summarise these points in Boxes 2.3 and 2.4 and give full details on writing a protocol in Chapter 3.

BOX 2.3 SUMMARY

Reasons for writing a research protocol

Scientific Focuses ideas about the research question; sets it in context of what is already known.

Feasibility Sample size calculations and statistical plan help to ensure that aims can be achieved.

Monitoring Provides a timetable and plan to monitor the progress of the study.

Organisational Provides the basis for applications for funding and ethical approval.

Aide memoire for writing up the study at a later date.

BOX 2.4 SUMMARY

Summary of a research protocol

◆ Title

◆ Abstract

◆ Purpose of the study; aims

◆ Background

◆ Study design

◆ Justification for sample size

◆ Plan of statistical analysis

◆ Ethical issues

◆ Costs

◆ Timetable

◆ Personnel

2.3 Data collection

The collection of data—what is actually collected and the format it is in—is obviously related to the study protocol. It is important to know in advance what we are going to do with the data in order to ensure that it is collected in the right format. For example, if we want to calculate mean age in a study group then we should record actual age rather than age in 10 year age bands.

BOX 2.5 INFORMATION

Points concerning using existing datasets

- Can be cheaper and quicker than collecting new data

- The research question needs to be defined and researched in the same way as for a primary study

- A clear analysis plan is needed to avoid over-analysing the data

- Note that the dataset may not contain all the necessary information to answer the new question

- Where data are analysed that have been collected for another purpose, this is sometimes referred to as **secondary analysis**

BOX 2.6 INFORMATION

Beware of collecting too much data

Why are you collecting it?
Will it actually be analysed?

Disadvantages of long questionnaires are:

- They may discourage people from taking part and so lower the response rate

- Questions may be answered less carefully

- Data processing time may be increased and results may be delayed

- They may lead to multiple hypothesis tests which increase the chance of spurious significance

- Time and money may be wasted

However, it is important to collect what you do need as it may be difficult to get it later.

It may be possible to answer a research question using existing data (Box 2.5). When collecting original data, it is not always easy to know exactly which data to collect. We discuss some of the issues surrounding this in Box 2.6.

2.4 Transferring the data to computer: coding and data entry

The researcher needs to decide how the data are to be recorded. Before non-numeric data from a questionnaire or data collection form are entered on to a computer, the responses need to be coded. That is, a unique number should be assigned to each possible response to facilitate statistical analysis. Some statistical packages will analyse data which is non-numeric, but in general it is easier to assign a different number to the different responses. For example, in Figure 2.1 the question 'When did you have rhinitis?' can be answered 'Dry season' ($=1$), 'Wet season' ($=2$), or 'Anytime' ($=3$).

The coding for this single question and coding for a multiple question are shown in Box 2.7. If data need coding, it can be useful to leave room on the data collection form or questionnaire for the codes to be added by the researcher after the form has been returned. These are sometimes in a column down the right-hand side of forms and labelled 'For office use only'. When data are coded, a coding schedule which describes what each code means should be kept for future reference.

Missing data are undesirable in any study. It may be important to be able to distinguish between data which are missing because the subject failed to respond, i.e. missed the question out completely, or where the answer was 'don't know'. For example, if doctors are asked about the management of a particular condition, they may give an answer or say that they don't know. This has a different meaning by allowing 'don't know' as a valid answer and assigning it a separate code from answers which are truly missing. A blank is often used to show a completely missing response, although it may be useful to use a particular code which is not a valid code for the other answers (e.g. 9) so that a numerical value is entered onto the computer for every variable.

It is important for the data collection forms to include a unique identifier for each subject so that, if needed, the computer records can be compared later with the original written forms. To maintain patient confidentiality, the patient identifier should not be a name or hospital number which might reveal the subject's identity. Data can be entered directly on to a computer using a spreadsheet (see Fig. 2.1). Each subject should have one line on the spreadsheet and each unique question should have one column. Some software will not accept variable names more than eight characters long, and spaces within variable names are not generally allowed. The first character of the name should be a letter, not a number, although numbers can go anywhere else (e.g. 'pulse1'). A record of the meaning of the variable names should be kept with the coding schedule.

Repeat measures should be given similar but unique names (e.g., 'diast1' 'diast2'). Note that there are no gaps in the rows and columns, and only one row is used for the variable names. Where the subjects are in several groups, all data should be in one spreadsheet, rather than several, with the group identity indicated in a separate column. If data are entered or stored in this format, then they will be much easier to transfer into a statistical package.

Data collection forms can be designed with specialised software, such as TeleForm (www. formrecognition.com) so that they can be scanned directly into the computer when completed (see Fig. 2.2). This may save time but is not entirely trouble free as the scanner may misread data if responses are slightly out of alignment or the handwriting is unclear. Tick boxes usually scan correctly but hand-written numbers may not. For example, a badly written 7 can look like a 9 and lead to scanning errors. Hence some checking is still needed when scanning is used.

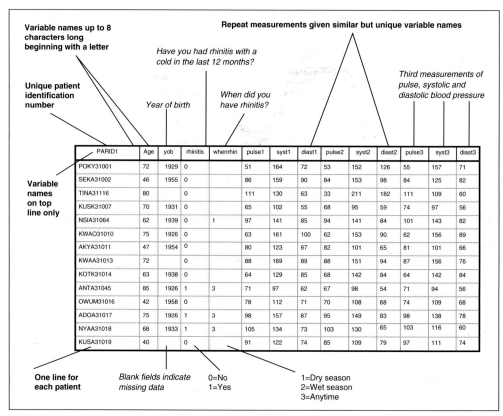

PARID1	Age	yob	rhinitis	whenrhin	pulse1	syst1	diast1	pulse2	syst2	diast2	pulse3	syst3	diast3
POKY31001	72	1929	0		51	164	72	53	152	126	55	157	71
SEKA31002	46	1955	0		86	159	90	84	153	98	84	125	82
TINA31116	80		0		111	130	63	33	211	182	111	109	60
KUSK31007	70	1931	0		65	102	55	68	95	59	74	97	56
NSIA31064	62	1939	0	1	97	141	85	94	141	84	101	143	82
KWAO31010	75	1926	0		63	161	100	62	153	90	62	156	89
AKYA31011	47	1954	0		80	123	67	82	101	65	81	101	66
KWAA31013	72		0		88	169	89	88	151	94	87	156	76
KOTK31014	63	1938	0		64	129	85	68	142	84	64	142	84
ANTA31045	85	1926	1	3	71	97	62	67	98	54	71	94	56
OWUM31016	42	1958	0		78	112	71	70	108	68	74	109	68
ADOA31017	75	1926	1	3	98	157	87	95	149	83	98	138	78
NYAA31018	68	1933	1	3	105	134	73	103	130	65	103	116	60
KUSA31019	40		0		91	122	74	85	109	79	97	111	74

Variable names up to 8 characters long beginning with a letter

Repeat measurements given similar but unique variable names

Have you had rhinitis with a cold in the last 12 months?

Unique patient identification number

Third measurements of pulse, systolic and diastolic blood pressure

When did you have rhinitis?

Year of birth

Variable names on top line only

One line for each patient

Blank fields indicate missing data

0=No
1=Yes

1=Dry season
2=Wet season
3=Anytime

Figure 2.1 Portion of a spreadsheet showing data collected from participants in a screening survey (example)

BOX 2.7 EXAMPLE

Coding single and multiple questions

1. The following **single question** was asked in the screening survey (see Fig 2.1)

When did you have rhinitis?
(*Please tick*)
☐ Dry season (=1)
☐ Wet season (=2)
☐ Anytime (=3)

The question would be coded 1, 2 or 3 according to the single answer given.

2. The following **multiple question** was asked in a study of patients with low back pain.

What did you expect from your consultation with your GP (Please tick all that apply)?
☐ *Prescription*
☐ *Advice*
☐ *Referral for x-ray*
☐ *Referral to consultant*
☐ *Certificate off work*

Although this is one question each person may tick a number of options. This needs to be entered as five separate variables each coded as 'no' or 'yes', which could be entered as 0 or 1

2.5 Data checking and cleaning

It is advisable to check the data as the study progresses rather than leave it until the end, as early checks may reveal problems which can be resolved. The process of data checking and cleaning involves looking for unlikely or impossible values or outliers, for example 'diast2 = 182', a very high value for diastolic blood pressure which should be checked (Fig. 2.3). Possible errors like this can be identified if summary statistics and/or a histogram of the data are produced (Fig. 2.4). In some data entry programmes, the user can set acceptable limits for each variable and thus force the computer to flag or reject values outside that range. If there is no evidence of a mistake and the value is plausible, then it should not be altered. For a fuller discussion of outliers see Altman (1991, Chapter 7).

Errors can also occur where the data have been incorrectly entered but the value entered is a possible value, and so is not flagged. This sort of error is very hard to detect. Entering the data twice, 'double entry', can minimise errors, although errors due to ambiguity in hand-writing may be entered wrongly twice. To look for these sorts of mistakes, we can hand-check a sample of forms to estimate the extent of any

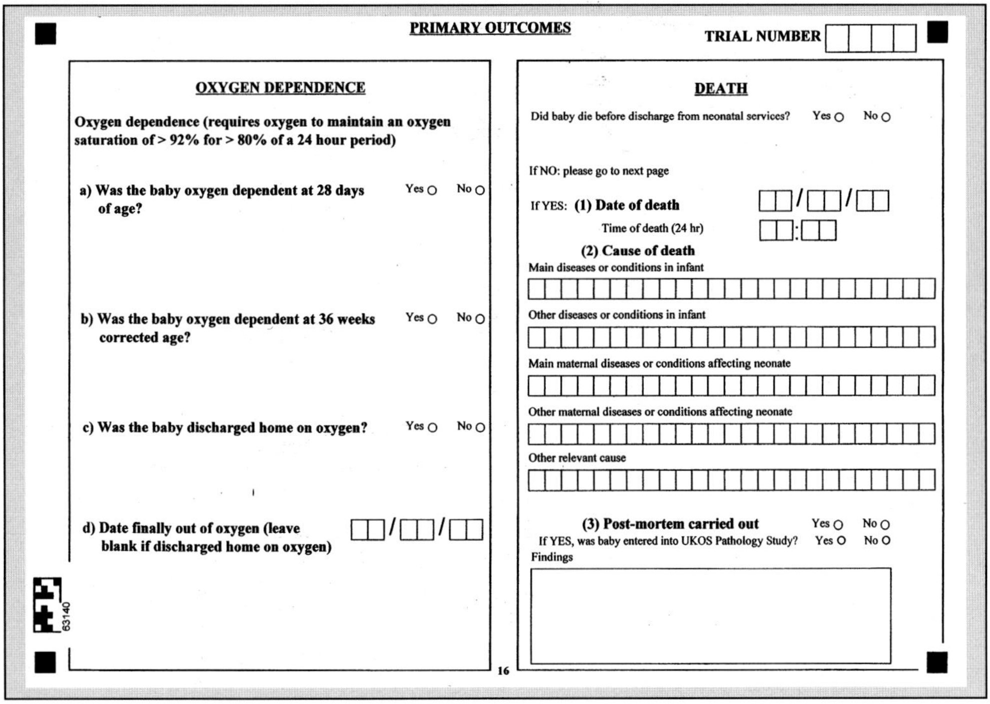
PRIMARY OUTCOMES
TRIAL NUMBER ☐☐☐

OXYGEN DEPENDENCE

Oxygen dependence (requires oxygen to maintain an oxygen saturation of > 92% for > 80% of a 24 hour period)

a) Was the baby oxygen dependent at 28 days of age? Yes ○ No ○

b) Was the baby oxygen dependent at 36 weeks corrected age? Yes ○ No ○

c) Was the baby discharged home on oxygen? Yes ○ No ○

d) Date finally out of oxygen (leave blank if discharged home on oxygen) ☐☐/☐☐/☐☐

DEATH

Did baby die before discharge from neonatal services? Yes ○ No ○

If NO: please go to next page

If YES: (1) Date of death ☐☐/☐☐/☐☐

Time of death (24 hr) ☐☐:☐☐

(2) Cause of death

Main diseases or conditions in infant

Other diseases or conditions in infant

Main maternal diseases or conditions affecting neonate

Other maternal diseases or conditions affecting neonate

Other relevant cause

(3) Post-mortem carried out Yes ○ No ○

If YES, was baby entered into UKOS Pathology Study? Yes ○ No ○

Findings

63140

16

Figure 2.2 Example of a form that can be scanned

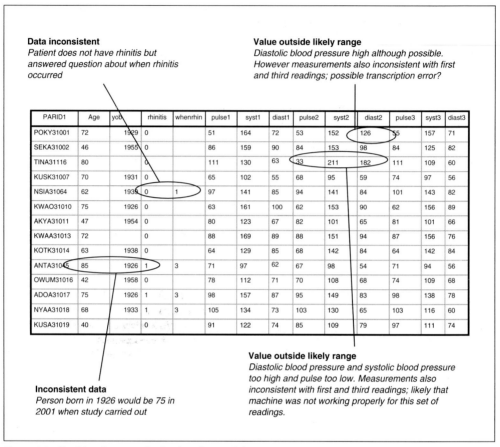

Data inconsistent
Patient does not have rhinitis but answered question about when rhinitis occurred

Value outside likely range
Diastolic blood pressure high although possible. However measurements also inconsistent with first and third readings; possible transcription error?

PARID1	Age	yob	rhinitis	whenrhin	pulse1	syst1	diast1	pulse2	syst2	diast2	pulse3	syst3	diast3
POKY31001	72	1929	0		51	164	72	53	152	126	55	157	71
SEKA31002	46	1955	0		86	159	90	84	153	98	84	125	82
TINA31116	80		0		111	130	63	33	211	182	111	109	60
KUSK31007	70	1931	0		65	102	55	68	95	59	74	97	56
NSIA31064	62	1939	0	1	97	141	85	94	141	84	101	143	82
KWAO31010	75	1926	0		63	161	100	62	153	90	62	156	89
AKYA31011	47	1954	0		80	123	67	82	101	65	81	101	66
KWAA31013	72		0		88	169	89	88	151	94	87	156	76
KOTK31014	63	1938	0		64	129	85	68	142	84	64	142	84
ANTA31045	85	1926	1	3	71	97	62	67	98	54	71	94	56
OWUM31016	42	1958	0		78	112	71	70	108	68	74	109	68
ADOA31017	75	1926	1	3	98	157	87	95	149	83	98	138	78
NYAA31018	68	1933	1	3	105	134	73	103	130	65	103	116	60
KUSA31019	40		0		91	122	74	85	109	79	97	111	74

Inconsistent data
Person born in 1926 would be 75 in 2001 when study carried out

Value outside likely range
Diastolic blood pressure and systolic blood pressure too high and pulse too low. Measurements also inconsistent with first and third readings; likely that machine was not working properly for this set of readings.

Figure 2.3 Checking for errors in the data (example)

problems. If problems appear to be present, then further hand-checking, particularly for key variables, is advisable. This is another reason why it is a good idea to do some quality checks early on in the study.

Another type of data error is internal inconsistency, for example, 'rhinitis = 0' ('no rhinitis') and 'whenrhin = 1' ('have rhinitis in the dry season'). This was noticed when the data were cross-tabulated. In some cases it may not be obvious which responses are correct. Where there is doubt, it is advisable to discuss the options with another team member and/or the statistician who will analyse the data.

2.6 Using computer packages

Many commercially produced statistical packages are available such as Stata, SPSS, SAS, S-Plus, Minitab, and countless more. The choice of which to use will depend on your budget, on what analyses

you want to do, and to some extent on your personal preferences. There are also public domain statistical programs and spreadsheets that are available free or at minimal cost (Box 2.8). Some of these will calculate confidence intervals from summary data. This may be particularly useful for SPSS users since SPSS does not always give confidence intervals (e.g. a confidence interval for a single proportion).

In this book we will demonstrate the use of Stata and SPSS for statistical analyses. In addition, we will use Epi-Info for sample-size calculations. Boxes 2.8 and 2.9 list the main features of each of these and a few other selected programs.

Menu-driven programs provide the user with a list of possibilities to choose from, selected by 'point and click' if the program is MS Windows based. Many users like selecting from menus since it does not require them to learn the syntax of commands. The disadvantages of menu-driven programs include their inflexibility, their relative slowness if a

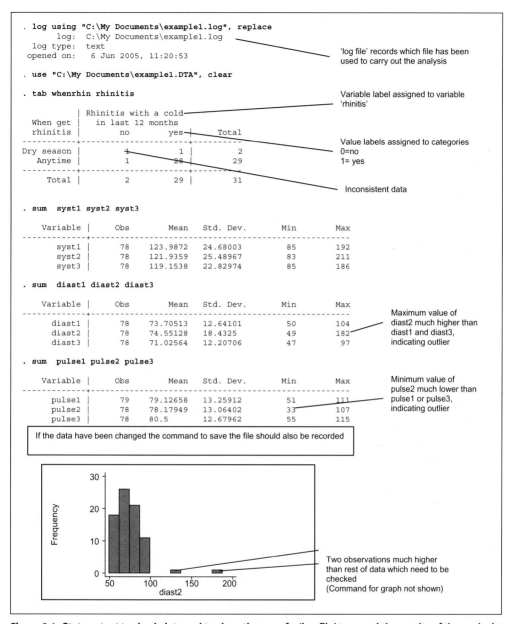

```
. log using "C:\My Documents\example1.log", replace
        log:  C:\My Documents\example1.log
   log type:  text
  opened on:    6 Jun 2005, 11:20:53

. use "C:\My Documents\example1.DTA", clear

. tab whenrhin rhinitis

            | Rhinitis with a cold
  When get  |   in last 12 months
  rhinitis  |       no       yes        Total
------------+-----------------------+----------
 Dry season |        1         1             2
    Anytime |        1        28            29
------------+-----------------------+----------
      Total |        2        29            31

. sum  syst1 syst2 syst3

    Variable |       Obs        Mean    Std. Dev.        Min        Max
-------------+--------------------------------------------------------
       syst1 |        78    123.9872     24.68003         85        192
       syst2 |        78    121.9359     25.48967         83        211
       syst3 |        78    119.1538     22.82974         85        186

. sum   diast1 diast2 diast3

    Variable |       Obs        Mean    Std. Dev.        Min        Max
-------------+--------------------------------------------------------
      diast1 |        78    73.70513     12.64101         50        104
      diast2 |        78    74.55128      18.4325         49        182
      diast3 |        78    71.02564     12.20706         47         97

. sum  pulse1 pulse2 pulse3

    Variable |       Obs        Mean    Std. Dev.        Min        Max
-------------+--------------------------------------------------------
      pulse1 |        79    79.12658     13.25912         51        111
      pulse2 |        78    78.17949     13.06402         33        107
      pulse3 |        78        80.5     12.67962         55        115
```

'log file' records which file has been used to carry out the analysis

Variable label assigned to variable 'rhinitis'

Value labels assigned to categories
0=no
1= yes

Inconsistent data

Maximum value of diast2 much higher than diast1 and diast3, indicating outlier

Minimum value of pulse2 much lower than pulse1 or pulse3, indicating outlier

If the data have been changed the command to save the file should also be recorded

Two observations much higher than rest of data which need to be checked
(Command for graph not shown)

Figure 2.4 Stata output to check data and to show the use of a 'log file' to record the results of the analysis

complex procedure is required, and the difficulty of remembering how to repeat a complex analysis. Command-driven programs require the user to write commands according to a specific syntax in order to carry out the analysis. If the syntax is wrongly typed, the command will not execute.

Spreadsheets are very useful for entering and manipulating data, and some researchers use them for data analysis. In general we are cautious about

recommending this since the scope of the analyses tends to be limited unless specialist modules are added on.

It is good practice to write a statistical analysis plan at the outset of a study, to guide the analysis (see section 3.7). This will ensure that the analyses performed answer the original study questions and prevent multiple ad hoc analyses and spurious significant findings. Both Stata and SPSS produce

BOX 2.8 INFORMATION

Some software available on the www, free or at modest price

Epi-Info (www.cdc.gov)

- Written primarily for case–control studies but can be used with other designs
- Menu- or command-driven
- Will be used in this book for sample size calculations for proportions
- Also performs basic statistical analyses (not covered here)

Clinstat (www-users.york.ac.uk)

- Written by Martin Bland, York University
- DOS-based menu-driven program
- Basic statistical analysis from data or summary statistics
- Sample size calculations

Biconf (www-users.york.ac.uk)

- Written by Martin Bland, York University
- Exact confidence intervals for rates and proportions

CIPROPORTION (www.cardiff.ac.uk)

- Written by Robert Newcombe, Cardiff University
- Annotated Excel spreadsheets. The user enters their summary data

Confidence Interval analysis (www.som.soton.ac.uk)

- Accompanies the book *Statistics with Confidence* (Altman *et al.*2000)
- Book purchase required for license key

Stats Direct (www.statsdirect.com)

- Recently written for medical researchers
- Wide range of statistical analyses applicable to medicine
- Easy to use
- Emphasis on confidence intervals
- 10 day free trial

BOX 2.9 INFORMATION

Commercial programs illustrated in this book

Stata

- Widely used by statisticians and medical researchers
- Command driven and menu driven, Windows based
- Simple command structure
- Simple and complex analysis
- Sample size calculations for proportions and means

SPSS

- Widely used by social scientists and medical researchers
- Menu driven, Windows based
- Can run from commands but syntax is relatively complicated
- Simple and complex analysis
- Does not do sample size calculations

detailed results for many analyses and not all of these are appropriate to all situations. In this book we will show examples of many analyses and will indicate which results apply in particular situations. However, we advise researchers to be careful and to read the user manual if in any doubt or seek advice from an experienced user. It is important to check the assumptions underlying any statistical procedures, and only to report the results which you understand. If the assumptions which the analysis makes about the data are not true, then results may be invalid. Unfortunately, the computer may not warn you about this, and so it is all too easy to produce analyses which look fine but are in fact meaningless.

2.7 Record keeping

Good record keeping is an essential part of the statistical analysis. Records should be kept of data coding, checking, cleaning, and analysis, and the results (Box 2.10). Most programs will produce an electronic copy or log file of the results of the analyses. This file will record the names of the data files used, and the commands that have been run to make any changes to the data and to carry out the statistical analysis. An example using Stata is shown in Figure 2.4. Having a log file means that any analysis can easily be reproduced. This may save a lot of time if the analysis needs to be repeated, for example if an error is discovered in the data. In the rest of the book we will only show the parts of the log file relevant to the analysis being demonstrated.

BOX 2.10 HELPFUL TIPS

Good record keeping

+ Have a written coding schedule and record any amendments to it clearly and systematically

+ Record any changes made to individual participant data with an explanation if necessary e.g. *'impossible value, set to missing'*

+ Use a computer log file to record any changes made to the data on the computer (see Fig 2.4)

+ Use a computer log file as in Figure 2.4 to record the results of the analysis and commands used to produce the results

Remember that others may need to check or use your data, or check your research results at a later stage.

2.8 Presenting results

When we present results either orally or in writing, we want our audience or readers to be interested in and to understand the message we are giving. If our presentation is unclear or muddled or just too long, then we may lose our audience or readers. Hence we need to present results in a clear and logical way that communicates our findings.

The format of the presentation will depend on the medium we are using—written or oral. For example, we may use a graph or chart to show results in an oral presentation where we would use a table in a written document. We will be addressing these aspects in detail in Chapter 5.

2.9 When to seek help from a statistician

We advise researchers to consult a medical statistician early in the protocol development phase.

A medical statistician is able to help with design issues as well as perform sample size calculations and do chi-square tests! Some studies which appear to be straightforward may involve subtle design or analysis issues.

This is particularly true of randomised controlled trials which need to be rigorously carried out. Hence we suggest that advice on design and analysis is obtained at the planning stage. Other things that statisticians can advise on include questionnaire design, planning the analysis (to be done at the outset), writing up in general, and interpreting the results. If the study is complex, such as a large cohort study or a multi-centre clinical trial, then the research team should include a statistician to take part in actually running the study as well as taking responsibility for analysing the data.

Chapter summary

Key points when planning research

+ Define a research question that can be answered

+ Write a protocol at the outset

+ Seek statistical advice early on

+ Only collect data you really need

+ Enter data onto a computer in an appropriate format

+ Check data quality early on

+ Consider involving a statistician as a collaborator

Writing a research protocol

3.1 The development cycle

A good research protocol describes the details of, and the rationale for, the research study that is being proposed. This is not to be confused with a clinical treatment protocol (Box 3.1) which describes how patients should be managed. The main components of a research protocol are described in Chapter 2 (Box 2.4). In this chapter we will discuss the sample-size calculations and plan of statistical analysis in more detail. However, these aspects cannot be considered in isolation. Developing a protocol is often an iterative process, as initial ideas are thought through, problems identified, the question redefined, and so on. For example, a researcher may have a good idea, a sound study design, and a robust outcome measure, but having calculated the required sample size finds that the proposed study cannot be achieved in the available time and/or with the available resources. Alternatively, background reading may reveal that the chosen research question has already been answered, or that a proposed intervention is unlikely to have the desired effect (Box 3.2). It is far better to identify such problems at the outset than later on when trying to publish the study.

3.2 Title

The project should be given a title which clearly reflects the aims of the study. The title introduces the readers to the project and is the first indication the reader has about what the researcher is trying to do. Careful thought needs to be given to the title so that it is accurate, not too long, and intelligible to the

---

BOX 3.1 INFORMATION

How a research protocol differs from other protocols

Research protocol

- Why the study is being carried out

- What is to be done and by whom

- How the results are going to be analysed

Clinical protocol

- Clinical protocols or guidelines are used to determine good practice in different clinical situations, e.g. how patients should be managed

- May be part of a *research* protocol but is not sufficient in itself for a research study

Manual of operations

- For larger studies it may be advisable to write a fuller protocol after funding has been agreed giving the precise details of how the study is to be carried out and what to do in specific situations. This is sometimes referred to as a manual of operations.

BOX 3.2 EXAMPLE

Redefining a research aim

Aim 1

- *To reduce the number of miscarriages due to infection.*

This is not a research aim. It is doing something to improve health rather than finding something out.

Aim 2

- *To investigate whether screening and treating women for bacterial vaginosis reduces the chance of early miscarriage.*

This asks a question but may not be achievable since it would require a large, and therefore expensive, randomised controlled trial screening some women and not others. This would only be justified if there was sufficient evidence that bacterial vaginosis is associated with early miscarriage.

Aim 3

- *To determine if bacterial vaginosis detected before 10 weeks is associated with miscarriage before 16 weeks.*

This aim answers a question, and was achievable within the funding constraints and was appropriate to current knowledge.

---

non-specialist. Sometimes the title is included on a patient information sheet, in which case it will need to be written in relatively simple language.

3.3 Aims of the research study

A research protocol is analogous to a route planning map. We need to know where we are going (the aims) and have a broad view of how we are going to get there (the study design) but also include some finer details so that we know what to do at certain points on the journey (details such as recruitment procedures). We also need to justify why we are going there, especially if other people may be inconvenienced in the process (background). Unless we are clear about where we are going we cannot plan an efficient route. Similarly, without clear aims it is impossible to write a good research protocol.

Research is about finding out and asking questions. Research aims should clearly state what the project is aiming to find out. While the motive for research may be to improve the care of patients and this may be a worthwhile aim, it is not a research aim. This is illustrated in the example in Box 3.2. A clear statement of aims makes writing, reading, and reviewing a protocol much easier.

3.4 Primary and secondary aims

Sometimes researchers may want to answer several questions from one study. This is often because collecting the data is time consuming and expensive, and so the researchers want to make the best use of the data. However, there are drawbacks. If too many hypotheses are tested in a study, there is an increased chance of spurious statistical significance. For a fuller discussion of this see Bland (2000, Chapter 9). Altman (1991, Chapter 15) recommends

Primary and secondary aims—UKOS study

Primary aim

Does early intervention with high-frequency oscillatory ventilation reduce mortality and incidence of chronic lung disease among babies with gestational age <29 weeks compared with conventional ventilation?

Secondary aim

Does high-frequency oscillatory ventilation affect age at death, age at discharge, major cranial abnormality, air leak, failure of treatment, hearing, necrotizing enterocolitis, patent ductus arteriosus, postnatal systemic steroid use, pulmonary haemorrhage, and retinopathy of prematurity?

Study design

Randomised controlled trial.

Writing a protocol—study design

Type of study; most studies will be one of the following

♦ Intervention study (trial)—randomised or not

♦ Cohort study

♦ Cross–sectional survey

♦ Case–control study

Discuss reason for choice of design and its advantages and disadvantages.

Selection of subjects

♦ Define population

♦ How will subjects be selected? What sampling method will be used?

♦ Describe and justify recruitment procedures (are they feasible?)

♦ What steps are taken to ensure a high response rate?

♦ How many subjects will be required and how was this chosen?

♦ State inclusion and exclusion criteria

Data collection and analysis

♦ What data are to be collected and why?

♦ What factors are thought to affect the outcome?

♦ What factors may distort the representativeness of the findings?

♦ What are the outcome measures in the study?

♦ Is it possible to collect these data?

How will the data be collected and by whom?

♦ Questionnaires, interviews, or routine data sources?

♦ Have any questionnaires proposed been validated?

♦ Will staff training be required?

♦ What measures are taken to avoid bias (e.g. blinding among patients, assessors, and data analysts)?

How will the data be processed

♦ On a computer database?

♦ Will the data be validated?

♦ What steps have been taken to ensure data confidentiality?

---

that trials should only have one primary outcome and that other outcomes should be considered to be of secondary importance. This is illustrated by the UKOS trial (Box 3.3).

3.5 Study design

Box 3.4 outlines the main issues that need to be clarified when writing the study design section. This can then form the basis of the methods section when writing up the study.

3.6 Sample size calculations

We need to decide at the outset of a study how many subjects we are going to recruit. The study can then be costed and its feasibility assessed. The number of subjects should be large enough to avoid having inconclusive results and yet not so large that subjects are put to unnecessary inconvenience and the study becomes unnecessarily expensive.

There are several textbooks available which describe sample size calculations and give explanations of the terms involved (Altman 1991; Machin *et al.* 1997; Bland 2000; Petrie and Sabin 2000; www.sgul.ac.uk). The actual sample size calculations can be carried out by hand using a calculator, or using a diagram called a nomogram (Altman 1991; Petrie and Sabin 2000), or using books of tables

(Machin *et al.* 1997), or using a statistics package (e.g. Clinstat, Epi-Info (Box 2.8), Stata (Box 2.9)).

We will consider here only how to present the results of such calculations in the protocol with reference to output from Stata and Epi-Info. For simplicity, we will only consider the three most common scenarios: prevalence studies, studies comparing two proportions, and studies comparing two means.

3.6.1 Prevalence studies

Here we study one group of people and estimate the prevalence of a disease in that group. No comparisons are made and no significance tests are carried out, but we can specify the accuracy of our estimate of prevalence by calculating the confidence interval, usually the 95% confidence interval. This is a range of values which has a 95% probability of containing the true population prevalence we are trying to estimate.

Box 3.5 lists the information required to do the calculations. These can be done in Epi-Info. Box 3.6 gives an example of a sample size statement from a survey of women to estimate the prevalence of chlamydia infection. All the assumptions made are contained in the sample size statement and prior information is referenced. Figure 3.1 shows the

---

BOX 3.5 INFORMATION

Information required for sample size calculations for estimating a prevalence with a certain accuracy

An estimate of the size of prevalence expected. This can be obtained from pilot studies or published studies. If there is no information available use 0.50 or 50% which will tend to be conservative, i.e. overestimate the sample size.

Confidence level. This is usually set to 95% but can be 90% or 99%.

Required width of the confidence interval. The researcher decides how precise the estimate is to be and this determines how wide the interval must be. The accuracy will usually be half the width of the interval. For example, in estimating a percentage expected to be close to 40%, the researcher may decide that this should be accurate to within 2 percentage points, i.e. ±2 percentage points. Thus the width of the confidence interval will be 4 percentage points.

BOX 3.6 EXAMPLE

Sample size statement for chlamydia prevalence study

Chlamydia study

Aim

To calculate the prevalence of chlamydia infection among women attending the GP for cervical smears.

Information required

- Estimate of the prevalence = 7% (from previous studies)
- Confidence level = 95% (decided by the researcher)
- Accuracy of ±1.4 percentage points (decided by the researcher)

Required sample size

1300 women (from Epi-Info).

Sample size statement

1300 women would allow estimation of the prevalence of chlamydia infection to within 1.4 percentage points either side of the estimated prevalence using a 95% confidence interval, assuming that the prevalence is approximately 7%.

(Oakeshott *et al.* 1998)

The estimate of prevalence came from unpublished data from another researcher.

---

output from Epi-Info related to this calculation. The number of subjects was rounded up from 1276 to 1300 in the protocol.

Note that Epi-Info expects the prevalence to be entered as a percentage (proportions multiplied by 100), whereas Stata expects proportions.

3.6.2 Screening studies (sensitivity and specificity)

Studies to estimate sensitivity and specificity are also based on proportions but have the added complication that each proportion will be calculated using only part of the sample. The number of subjects for the sensitivity calculation is the number of true positives and the number of subjects for the specificity is the number of true negatives. If the expected number of true positives is low, then even if the total sample is large the estimate of the sensitivity may be imprecise and thus have a wide confidence interval.

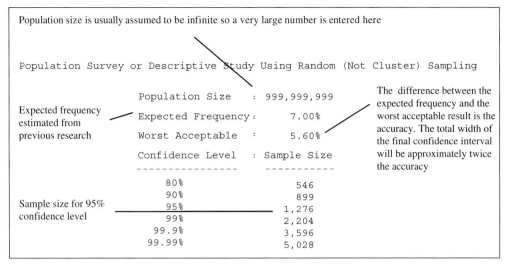

Population size is usually assumed to be infinite so a very large number is entered here

Population Survey or Descriptive Study Using Random (Not Cluster) Sampling

Expected frequency estimated from previous research

```
             Population Size    :  999,999,999
             Expected Frequency :      7.00%
             Worst Acceptable   :      5.60%
             Confidence Level   :  Sample Size
             ----------------      ----------
                  80%                  546
                  90%                  899
                  95%                1,276
                  99%                2,204
                  99.9%              3,596
                  99.99%             5,028
```

The difference between the expected frequency and the worst acceptable result is the accuracy. The total width of the final confidence interval will be approximately twice the accuracy

Sample size for 95% confidence level

Figure 3.1 Output for sample size for a prevalence from Epi-Info

Where the true status of the patients is not known in advance, the prevalence will also need to be estimated. This is illustrated by a cohort study to test a non-invasive antenatal screening method for chromosomal abnormalities (Box 3.7). The true status of the baby may not be known until birth, and so all babies would need to be screened and followed up to see which of those that test positive were really affected. The prevalence of chromosomal abnormalities is very low, so even with a large sample there will be few babies who are true positives from which to estimate the sensitivity. It may be that we have to accept wide confidence intervals, but it is useful to know the limitations of the study in advance.

3.6.3 Comparison studies

We may wish to compare two or more groups of subjects. The outcome might be either a proportion or a mean. Here we need to consider what kind of difference is of such clinical significance that we would not want our study to be non-significant if this difference really existed in the whole population. The information required in order to carry out the calculation is given in Boxes 3.8 and 3.10.

3.6.4 Computer packages

Stata will do either a difference of means or a difference of proportions. Epi-Info will only compare

---

BOX 3.7 EXAMPLE

Sample size for sensitivity

Aim

To calculate the sensitivity and specificity of nuchal translucency screening for chromosomal abnormalities using an unselected cohort of pregnant women.

Information required

- Estimate of the prevalence of chromosomal abnormalities = 1% (from previous studies)
- Estimate of sensitivity = 70% (from previous studies)
- Confidence level = 95% (decided by the researcher)
- Accuracy of ±20 percentage points (decided by the researcher)

Required sample size

20 babies with chromosomal abnormalities (1% or 0.01 of population) and hence 2000 pregnant women required overall (20/0.01).

Sample size statement

2000 pregnant women are likely to have 20 babies with chromosomal abnormalities. This would allow the sensitivity of the test to be estimated to within ±20 percentage points using a 95% confidence interval assuming that the sensitivity is approximately 70%.

Information required to compare two proportions

Estimate of proportion in one group. Can be obtained from pilot studies, other publications.

Significance level. Usually set to 5%, but sometimes 1% or lower.

Power. The probability of detecting a specified size of effect if it exists. Power usually set to 80% or 90%.

The smallest effect of interest. This needs to be decided by the researcher. It is the size of effect that is clinically important. This may be a difference of proportions (risk difference), relative risk, or odds ratio.

The ratio of the numbers of subjects in each group. For most randomised trials this will be 1, i.e. the groups will all be the same size but group sizes may be very different in observational studies (e.g. comparing smokers and non-smokers where there are more non-smokers than smokers in the population).

Sample size statement for comparing two proportions

UKOS study

Aim

To compare prevalence of death or chronic lung disease in premature babies randomised to two methods of ventilation.

Outcome

Death or chronic lung disease at 36 weeks post menstrual age.

Information required

- Estimate of the prevalence in control group = 67% (from previous studies)
- Significance level = 5% (decided by the researcher)
- Risk difference to be detected 11 percentage points (i.e. 56% in intervention group)
- Power 90% (decided by researcher)
- Babies will be randomised to two equal-sized groups

Required sample size

428 babies in each group (from Stata).

Sample size statement

428 babies in each group would allow a difference of 11 percentage points in the prevalence of death or chronic lung disease at 36 weeks post menstrual age, assuming that the prevalence is 67% in the control group with a power of 90%, using a 5% significance level (Johnson *et al.* 2002).

Note: This example has been simplified here for illustration. The UKOS study actually considered a range of possible sample sizes from 800 to 1200 since it was uncertain at the outset how many babies could be recruited in the time available. The paper reports this in detail and also gives a full justification of the control group prevalence (see Chapter 12 for details).

percentages. Examples of output from both packages are given in Figures 3.2–3.4. Stata expresses power and significance levels as proportions, but power is normally expressed as a percentage in sample size statements. Epi-Info expresses significance as the confidence level, which is 100—significance. Therefore if the required significance level is 5%, then 95% is entered into the 'confidence' box in Epi-Info (Fig. 3. 3).

3.6.5 Sample size for two proportions

The power is related to the minimum difference between the two proportions, expressed as a risk difference, relative risk, or odds ratio. Stata requires the user to specify the two proportions which make up that difference, not the difference (Fig. 3.2). Epi-Info is more flexible and requires one percentage and then either the second percentage or the relative risk or odds ratio (Fig. 3.3).

Box 3.8 summarises the information required to carry out a sample size calculation for comparing two proportions. Box 3.9 shows an example of a sample size statement to compare two proportions

taken from a randomised controlled trial comparing two methods of ventilation in babies. The calculations can be done in either Stata or Epi-Info and are shown in Figures 3.2 and 3.3.

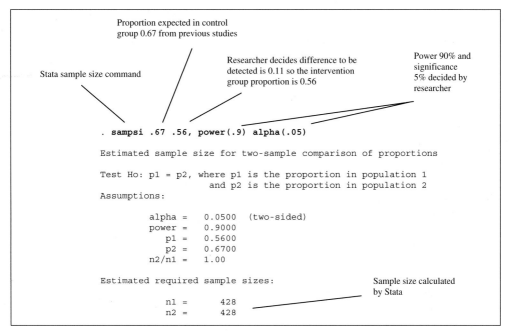

Figure 3.2 Output for sample size for two proportions from Stata

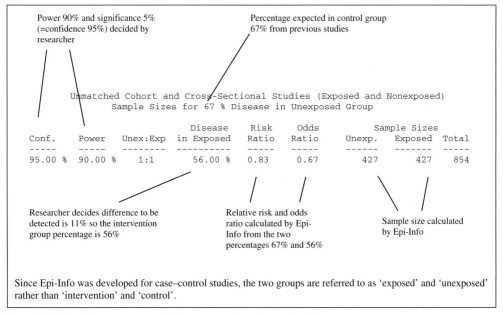

Figure 3.3 Output for sample size for two proportions from Epi-Info

3.6.6 **Sample size for two means**

Box 3.10 shows the information required to carry out a sample size calculation to compare two means. Instead of an estimate of the prevalence in one group an estimate of the standard deviation is required. The calculations can be done in Stata but not in Epi-Info. When calculating sample sizes for the difference between two means, Stata requires both means to be given (Fig. 3.4). However, the absolute value of the means does not matter, only the difference between them. In the birthweight example, the same sample size would be obtained when the two means were 2000 and 2180. This is not true for proportions, where the sample size depends not only on the difference but also on the absolute value of the proportions.

Box 3.11 gives an example of a sample size statement from a study comparing mean birthweight in two groups. The output for Stata is given in Figure 3.4. Note that in this example, the calculated sample size was multiplied up because the study wanted to be able to detect differences between social class subgroups which were only 10% of the total sample. Hence if the 10% subgroup needed to contain 163 subjects, then the total sample size needed to be 1630.

3.6.7 **Unequal-sized groups**

In most randomised controlled trials the treatment groups are equal in size. This is the most efficient design. However this is not always possible. If the ratio of subjects in one group to the other is not equal ie not 1.0, then the sample size calculations can still be done by specifying this ratio. In Stata this is done by adding an extra command to the **sampsi** statement. So if the required ratio was 9, then **r(9)** would be added to the command line after the comma (see Fig 3.4). Epi- Info also allows calculations with unequal sample sizes.

If we do not know how many subjects fall into each group, it is useful to carry out a sensitivity

---

BOX 3.11 EXAMPLE

Sample size statement for comparing two means

Birthweight study

Aim

To compare mean birthweight of babies in different social class subgroups.

Outcome

Birthweight.

Information required

- ◆ Estimate of the standard deviation of birthweight = 500g (from previous studies)
- ◆ Significance level = 5% (decided by the researcher)
- ◆ Difference to be detected 180g
- ◆ Power 90% (decided by researcher)

Required sample size

163 women in each group (from Stata).

Sample size statement

The target sample size was 326. This sample size is sufficient to detect differences in mean birthweight of 180g between two social class subgroups, with power 90%. A 5% significance level was assumed and a standard deviation of 500g (Brooke *et al.* 1989).

Note: The study wanted to be able to detect differences in subgroups as small as 10% of the total sample and so the target sample size was multiplied by 10 to give a final target sample of 1630 women.

BOX 3.10 INFORMATION

Information required to compare two means

Estimate of standard deviation. Can be obtained from pilot studies, other publications.

Significance level. Usually set to 5%, but sometimes 1% or lower.

Power. The probability of detecting a specified size of effect if it exists. Usually set to 80% or 90%.

The smallest effect of interest. This is the difference between the groups that is clinically important and we do not want to overlook. The researcher needs to decide this.

The ratio of the numbers of subjects in each group. For most randomised trials this will be 1, i.e. the groups will all be the same size but group sizes may be very different in observational studies.

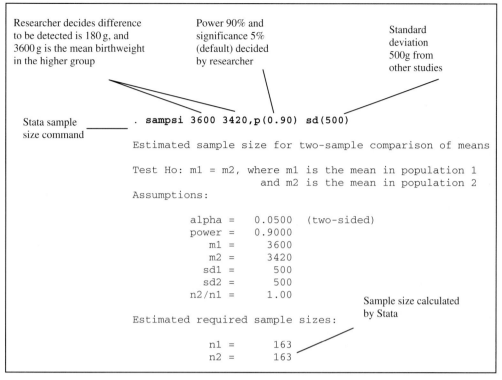

Figure 3.4 Output from Stata for sample size of the difference between two means

analysis on the sample size calculations and to recalculate the sample size using different assumptions.

3.6.8 Subgroup and multifactorial analyses

Sample size calculations for complex analyses such as multiple regression are not possible in Stata and Epi-Info and are not included in this book. A specialist package such as nQuery Advisor (www.statsolusa.com) is required. There are informal ways of dealing with these issues by calculating the sample size assuming a simple analysis will be performed but using a very high power such as 99%. However, we suggest that, to avoid under powered studies, advice is sought if such analyses are planned.

3.6.9 Cluster randomised trials

Most drug trials randomise individual participants to treatment groups. However, for trials investigating the effectiveness of different methods of health service delivery, whole groups (clusters) of individuals may be randomised. These are commonly known as cluster randomised trials. In the UK, general practices are often randomised as a cluster. If the clustering is ignored when the sample size calculations are done, the resultant number will be an underestimate of the true sample size required. In some cases the underestimation is substantial. Methods of calculating sample size for cluster trials are described by Kerry and Bland (1998a) and Donner and Klar (2000).

3.6.10 Presentation of sample size statements

Examples of sample size statements are given in Boxes 3.6, 3.7, 3.9, and 3.11. Where results from other studies have been used, these should be referenced. Any assumptions made should be clearly stated. It is important to state not only the power but also the difference to be detected. This is because as the difference to be detected increases so does the power of the study, for the same level of significance.

In Box 3.9 the sample size statement expresses the difference between the two percentages as '11 percentage points' difference, rather than 11% to avoid confusion. An 11% difference would imply 67% in one group and 60% in the other ($0.89 \times 0.67 \times 100$).

3.6.11 Feasibility

Along with the sample size statements, it is useful to give evidence of the feasibility of the planned sample size. In the UKOS study, the number of eligible babies normally admitted to a unit in a year was presented in the protocol to show that the target recruitment was feasible.

3.7 Plan of statistical analysis

An outline plan of statistical analysis should be presented in the protocol. There are several reasons for preparing the plan in advance. First, it identifies any problems with the analysis that might indicate that a different study design would be better. Secondly, by stating the main analysis in advance, it is known that these were preplanned. This protects against the possibility of the researcher changing the outcome or method of analysis when the first outcome or method did not give the anticipated or desired results. This gives the results more credibility and ensures that the study is fairly reported. Carrying out 100 different analyses and only reporting those which show significant findings gives a biased view of the results of the study. If the original research question is interesting and useful, then the results will be worth presenting regardless of whether they are significant or not, provided that the study has been properly carried out. What is of less interest is a poorly conducted study where conclusions cannot be drawn because of flaws in the study design or too small a sample size.

Sometimes, after looking at the data, the researcher decides that a certain comparison should be made or looks 'interesting'. This type of analysis is known as post hoc or data-driven analysis, and will always carry less weight than an analysis that is preplanned.

Box 3.12 shows the main points that should be covered in an analysis plan. The analysis plan for the early pregnancy study clearly states that the outcome is miscarriage before 16 weeks (Box 3.13). A secondary unplanned analysis of time of miscarriage was carried out when results showed no increase in miscarriage overall. This was inconsistent with other studies which had shown an increase in the second trimester. This new analysis was reported as a secondary analysis and given less weight in the reporting of the results.

BOX 3.12 INFORMATION
Plan of statistical analysis

- Distinguish between primary and secondary analyses
- State the outcomes to be analysed and the groups to be compared
- State methods of analysis, significance tests, and level of significance to be used
- State assumptions which need to be verified
- List confounders to be investigated and possibly adjusted for in a multifactorial model
- If there are several outcomes, describe the strategy for dealing with the possibility of spurious significant findings (type I errors)

3.8 Ethical approval

Medical research studies involving patients require approval from a research ethics committee. The responsibility of the committee is primarily to 'ensure that the research respects the rights, dignity, safety and well-being of the individual research participants' (www.dh.gov.uk).

The ethics committee also has a responsibility to ensure the scientific validity of the study as 'research which duplicates other work unnecessarily or which is not of sufficient quality to contribute something useful to existing knowledge is itself unethical' (www.dh.gov.uk).

We will describe the ethical review process in the UK and give guidance as to how to present the statistical aspects of the study. Whilst the details of the process are UK specific, the recommendations are applicable in other countries since similar questions are likely to be asked.

3.8.1 Ethical approval process in the UK

The procedure for ethical review in the UK is described in detail on the website of the Central Office for Research Ethics Committees (www.corec.org.uk). Since 1 April 2004 all research studies in the UK need full review by one research ethics committee (REC). At the time of writing, this will often be the committee associated with the institution where the research is to be carried out but need not be. The membership of the ethics committee

---

BOX 3.13 EXAMPLE

Analysis plan for the early pregnancy study

Aim To see if bacterial vaginosis detected before 10 weeks is associated with miscarriage before 16 weeks.

Study design Cohort study.

Primary outcome Miscarriage before 16 weeks.

Analysis plan

Primary analysis

The relative risk of miscarriage before 16 weeks with bacterial vaginosis before 10 weeks will be calculated. Cox regression will be used to adjust for variable gestational age at recruitment. $P < 0.05$ will be taken as significant.

Secondary analysis

The following risk factors for bacterial vaginosis will be investigated:

    Age less than 25
    Afro-Caribbean ethnic group
    Social class 3 to 5
    Single marital status
    Previous oral contraception
    Smoking
    History of termination
    History of miscarriage
    History of preterm birth
    Concurrent chlamydia infection

The prevalence of bacterial vaginosis in women with and without these risk factors will be estimated and compared using relative risks.

Technical note

A survival analysis approach was used in this study to allow the inclusion of all miscarriages before 16 weeks (Oakeshott *et al.* 2002).

---

covers a wide variety of disciplines and includes lay and medical members and people with expertise in research methodology. If a study has not been independently peer reviewed, then the ethics committee will require sufficient information to ensure scientific validity. All applications are subject to statistical review and failure to provide a clear protocol may delay the application.

In addition to the application form and protocol, researchers must submit their patient information sheet and consent form. The COREC website provides advice on producing these. We advise researchers to avoid medical jargon, to use simple language, and to remember that patients need to understand what is going to happen and what is different from their normal care. Patients should be clearly told that they can refuse to take part without giving a reason. Patients should also be told why the study is being carried out and what the researcher hopes to achieve from it. This may encourage them to take part. It is important that reasons are justifiable; otherwise patients will be recruited under false pretences.

At the time of writing, the application form is submitted electronically. Several questions relating to statistical aspects are included, such as whether a formal power calculation has been carried out, and this requires sufficient detail to allow the calculations to be replicated. If standard methods such as those described in this chapter are used, it is not necessary to give the formulae but sufficient information must be given for someone else to check the calculations (see Boxes 3.5, 3.8, and 3.10.). The example statements in this chapter (Boxes 3.6, 3.7, 3.9 and 3.11) will suffice. The form also asks which statistical methods will be used and requires the statistical analysis plan as described earlier in this chapter.

For intervention trials involving medicinal products, the researcher needs to obtain a EudraCT (European Clinical Trials Directive) number prior to applying for ethical approval, and the application will be allocated to an REC through the Central Allocation System. For further information see the COREC website or contact the local research ethics office.

3.9 **Where it goes wrong**

It is very disappointing to plan a study and then fail to obtain funding or ethical approval. Funding is often competitive and subject to political pressures and changes, and so it is difficult to give general advice on this. However, the advice given in this chapter should ensure that the statistical aspects of the study are clearly presented. Box 3.14 also gives some advice on choosing a source of funding.

When a study is rejected, there may be feedback from the reviewers. Reviewers may not always be right but we recommend that they are taken seriously. Before applying to another funding body, it is sensible to revise the protocol in the light of their comments. It may be necessary to present a stronger case or to clarify some aspects. The new proposal may go back to the same specialist reviewer even if the application goes to a different funding body.

BOX 3.14 HELPFUL TIPS

Choosing a funding source

- Is the subject for research within the priority areas for this source of funding?

- Is the amount of funding required appropriate for the total funds available from this funding source?

- Is the expertise of the team sufficient to carry out the work?

- Has sufficient background work been carried out for this study? (e.g. literature review, pilot studies, etc.)

Ethical approval on the other hand is not competitive. Studies are approved on their own merit and on the implications for patients. Box 3.15 outlines common pitfalls for researchers in gaining ethical approval that we have observed.

BOX 3.15 HELPFUL TIPS

Common reasons for delay in obtaining ethical approval

- Failure to describe the precise aims of the study and why you want to do it

- Failure to demonstrate that the study will add to existing knowledge

- Failure to justify the sample size chosen, or worse, not to specify the sample size at all

- Poor explanation of sample size calculations so that they cannot be reproduced

- Unclear and/or inadequate information sheet. This is the most common reason for delayed approval

Chapter summary

Checklist for writing a research protocol

- The aims of the research project need to be clearly written and understood by a wide variety of people

- Sample size calculations are necessary to ensure results will be useful without putting too many people to unnecessary inconvenience or incurring unnecessary expense

- Assumptions of the calculations need to be explained and referenced where appropriate

- Writing a plan of the statistical analysis at the outset helps to ensure that the aims of the study can be fulfilled and protects the validity of the results

- The role of the ethics committee is primarily to protect patients' welfare, but it also has a responsibility towards the scientific validity of the study

Writing up a research study

4.1 Introduction

A research study report may be written for any one of several different purposes, with each requiring a specific format. Examples include an internal report, a report for a funding body or committee, a paper for a journal, a dissertation for an undergraduate or postgraduate degree or for one of the Royal Medical College examinations, or a thesis (e.g. MD, PhD). The general structure is mostly similar for all of these and follows the usual pattern for writing up the results of a scientific experiment: introduction, methods, results, and discussion (Box 4.1). (Exceptions are short reports and research letters, which we will discuss separately below.) The length and relative balance of each of these sections varies according to the purpose and specified format. For example, a paper for a journal will tend to be fairly short, often less than 3000 words, whereas a dissertation may be up to 20 000 words and a thesis considerably longer.

We outline below the contents of each of the sections of a research study report with particular reference to the statistical aspects.

4.2 Contents of each section of the report

4.2.1 Abstract

The main requirement for an abstract is that it should be brief and yet be a stand-alone document. It is the first thing that most people will read and, more importantly, may be all that is read if the reader has limited time or restricted access to the full document (e.g. when obtaining abstracts through online journals or databases).

BOX 4.1 INFORMATION

Basic structure of a scientific report

- ◆ Abstract
- ◆ Background
- ◆ Methods
- ◆ Results
- ◆ Discussion

BOX 4.2 EXAMPLE

Examples of required structures for abstracts

- ◆ **BMJ**—250 words maximum
  Objectives, design, setting, subjects, interventions, main outcome measures, results, conclusions

- ◆ **New England Journal of Medicine**—250 words maximum
  Background, methods, results, conclusion

- ◆ **University of London PhD**—300 words maximum
  No prescribed format

An abstract should state the purpose of the study and briefly describe the study design, the study subjects, and the variables measured. The results section should summarise the key findings on the main variables of interest and should provide estimates of sizes of effects with confidence intervals, wherever possible, as well as P values. Valid conclusions should be drawn without overstating or understating the interpretation of the findings. Common problems that we have observed include interpreting simple associations as causative, assuming that statistical significance implies clinical significance, and conversely assuming that 'not statistically significant' means that there is no effect or difference. Understating conclusions is less common, but some abstracts end with a statement along the lines 'the risk factor may be related to the disease', which probably could have been said without doing the study.

A structured abstract may be required with a specified work limit. Examples of specifications are given in Box 4.2, and Box 4.3 gives an example of a structured abstract.

BOX 4.3 EXAMPLE

Example of an abstract for a journal article

Objectives: To examine changes in the emergency workload of the London Ambulance Service (LAS) between 1989 and 1999.

Methods: All emergency responses by the LAS during week 16 in each of 1989, 1996 and 1999 were studied. For each week, 999 call responses were analysed by time and day of call, and age/sex of the patient. Call response rates were calculated using age/sex census population estimates for London. Changes in call rates over time were calculated as rate ratios.

Results: Emergency responses increased from 6624 to 13178 in the index weeks of 1989–1999. The ratio of response rates (1999/1989) was 1.91 (95% CI: 1.85,1.96). The proportion of out-of-hours calls increased significantly, from 68.8% in 1989 to 71.3% in 1999 ($P = 0.0003$). Response rates rose significantly more steeply for males than females from 1989–1999: rate ratio (95% CI); males 2.00 (1.91, 2.08), females 1.69 (1.62,1.77), $P<0.0001$. Response rates varied by age in each of the three years investigated. Rates were consistently highest for patients aged 75 and above, and lowest for those aged 5–14. However, there was no evidence that call rates had increased disproportionately in any particular age group ($P = 0.79$).

Conclusions: Demand for emergency ambulance services in London has doubled in a decade. This increase is similar for all age groups, with no evidence of a greater rise in demand among older people. Call rates have increased more steeply in men than in women. Demographic changes do not explain the observed increases in demand.

(Peacock *et al.* 2005)

4.2.2 Introduction

This sets the scene and describes the background to the study—what is already known about the topic, what are the gaps in knowledge, how the proposed study will add to this. In a journal article this section is likely to be short but will be much more detailed in a dissertation, report or thesis.

4.2.3 **Methods**

This section aims to describe how the study was conducted in sufficient detail for another researcher to be able to repeat the study. However, in a journal article, as opposed to a dissertation or report, space is usually limited and it can be difficult to go into much detail. Recently, the use of online www supplements has helped to remedy this problem by allowing the brief details in a paper to be supplemented by fuller details online.

The methods section should include details of the setting or area where the study was conducted, the subjects included, the study design, technical details of any measurements made, the rationale for the chosen sample size, and the statistical methods used to analyse the data. Some studies use routine data, and so the description of the subjects may only need to state the time period (see Box 4.3).

In other situations, subjects may be selected according to set criteria or diagnoses, and these should be stated. Alternatively, the subjects may simply be an unselected series of available patients in a time period. However the data or subjects were selected, it is important to be able to demonstrate that the selection was done in a systematic way which will enable the study's findings to be generalised. Box 4.4 gives examples of describing the sample taken from the UKOS study.

BOX 4.4 EXAMPLE

Extract from a methods section describing the sample

Infants were eligible for the study if their gestational age was between 23 weeks and 28 weeks plus 6 days; if they were born in a participating centre; if they required endotracheal intubation from birth; and if they required ongoing intensive care. Infants were excluded if they had to be transferred to another hospital for intensive care shortly after birth or if they had a major congenital malformation.

(Johnson *et al.* 2002)

The description of the study design should include the type of study (e.g. cross-sectional survey, case–control, cohort, randomised controlled trial, etc.). For case–control studies, the method of choosing controls and the definition of cases should be described. If cases are matched to controls, the method of matching should be described in sufficient detail to explain exactly how the controls were chosen. For example, 'cases were one-to-one matched to within 2 years using the general practice age/sex register'.

Where formal sample size calculations have been done, these should be reported (see Box 4.5), and where they are inappropriate or not possible, it is helpful to say so. Sometimes the original sample size estimates proved to be unachievable and therefore modified estimates are made. Box 4.5 gives examples of different scenarios.

Chapter 3 describes how to report sample size statements in a protocol, and the same principles apply to reporting in a paper. Further discussion of reporting sample size for a randomised clinical trial is given in Chapter 12.

The report should state any statistical methods used and, if appropriate, underlying assumptions. It is not enough simply to say that a particular statistical package was used, 'the data were analysed using SPSS' or that 'parametric methods were used', although the statistical package or software used

---

BOX 4.5 EXAMPLE

Examples of statements on sample size

◆ *No formal calculation but justification given*
This study was designed to be descriptive rather than analytical . . . a sample size of about 100 was feasible within the time available and was judged to be adequate to give reasonable numbers in the various categories of response expected. (Bruce *et al.* 2001)

◆ *Formal calculation*
The study aimed to recruit 800 babies. Assuming power of 0.9 and significance level 0.05, this was sufficient to detect a difference of 11 percentage points between treatment groups overall. (Johnson *et al.* 2002)

◆ *Formal calculation, later modified*
A pulmonary function subset sample size of 100 infants . . . would have enabled detection of a difference of 0.56 standard deviations between the groups, with 80% power at the 5% significance level. The achieved sample size fell below this target and allowing for unequal group sizes, enabled detection of 0.65 standard deviations between the groups. (Thomas *et al.* 2004)

should be specified. If the statistical method is not a standard technique, then a reference should be given. In a longer report there is room to give a full justification of the methods used. Box 4.6 gives a detailed example. The report of the statistical analysis clearly states the main outcome and the predictor variables and describes the type of data— here categorical data in three and two categories, respectively. Then the actual analysis (chi-square test for trend and logistic regression) is stated. Finally, we are told how the results will be presented (odds ratios and 95% confidence intervals) and what statistical package was used.

Further examples of how to describe specific statistical methods are given throughout the book.

Sometimes the researcher may not know in advance exactly which methods will be used as it can depend on early findings. In such circumstances it

is not obvious whether to include these methods in the methods section, as if they were determined in advance, or to describe them in the results section. We advise that the methods are described in the methods section if at all possible, unless the text flows better with them included with the results.

4.2.4 Results

The results section should begin by describing the study population. This should include the total numbers of subjects or observations, with a breakdown of these numbers to show the reasons for missing data (e.g. refusal, non-response, drop-out, data not recorded, etc.). The basic characteristics of the study population should be described. If the study is comparing groups, as in a randomised trial, then baseline data for the two groups should be given. If there is much information, is can be easier for the reader if it is presented in a table. Where there are many baseline variables, the choice of which to present is a matter of judgement. In Box 4.7 we give an example of summarising a subset of data from a larger sample. We had previously used this as a teaching exercise to illustrate how different types of data can be incorporated into just one table. (In the past we had noticed that new students and researchers tended to put each variable in a separate table, which not only wasted space but also made the results rather disjointed.) We provide guidelines on how to describe baseline characteristics in Chapter 5.

The main results of statistical analyses can often be summarised in tables and graphs. Missing data should be accounted for wherever possible so that the numbers 'add- up'. Often totals will vary from table to table by a small amount either because data are missing for that variable or because subjects do not answer a particular question. In such cases it is usually sufficient to give the maximum total and then to say 'numbers vary slightly from table to table owing to missing data'.

It is often easier to assimilate several numbers presented when they are in tables rather than if they are given in the text. This is certainly possible when writing a report or a dissertation or thesis where there is usually space to include many tables. However, this may not be possible when writing a journal article, as there may be a limit to the number of tables allowed. The text itself should describe and summarise the important features in terms of the sizes of effects, the differences between groups, the strengths of associations, etc., as appropriate. It is unnecessary to repeat information already given in tables, such as giving a

---

BOX 4.6 EXAMPLE

Describing the statistical methods

Description of study

This example comes from a study which aimed to investigate the association between self-reported domestic violence and health in primary school children. The survey consisted of a self-completion questionnaire.

The main outcome was self-reported exposure to domestic violence in three categories. The predictor variables were aspects of health care use, health behaviour, and social support.

Description of statistical analysis

The outcome was self-reported physical violence at home in the last month, with three categories of exposure: 'none', 'once or twice', and 'often'. The health outcomes included questions on health care use, health-related behaviours, and social support and were analysed as binary variables.

The chi-square test for trend was used to analyse the differences in proportions of health-related outcomes in the three violence exposure categories. Multivariable logistic regression was used to investigate the association between violence and health outcomes, after adjustment for socio-economic status. Results are presented as unadjusted and adjusted odds ratios with 95% confidence intervals. Data were analysed using Stata and in-house software.

(Stewart *et al.* 2004)

Baseline characteristics of a sample

Characterisics of study group: 230 pregnant women who missed antenatal clinic appointments

Variable	No.	Mean(SD) or %
Age (years)	229	26.1 (5.5)
Height (cm)	225	161.6 (6.3)
Weight (kg)	225	61.7 (10.4)
Alcohol (g/week)	230	17.3 (33.6)
Birthweight of baby (g)	229	3280 (477)
Marital status		
Married	156	69%
Single	59	26%
Windowed/separated /divorced	12	5%
Total	227	100%
Social class		
Non-manual	90	43%
Manual	117	57%
Total	207	100%
Education		
Minimum	137	61%
More than minimum	88	39%
Total	225	100%
Current smoking		
Smoker	118	52%
Non-smoker	110	48%
Total	228	100%

Possible statistical issues for inclusion in the discussion

- Size of effects observed, width of CIs
- Consequences of multiple testing
- Limitations of methods of analysis
- Limitations due to design, e.g. interpretation of non-randomised intervention studies
- Known and unknown confounding
- Effects of missing data
- Accuracy of measurements made—random error/bias
- Future work, new data, further analyses

Example of the statistical interpretation of results in the discussion section

Our findings were of greater magnitude than those observed by Hoek and others . . . (who) reported a 3% increase . . . our estimate was equivalent to a 13% increase in risk, but the 95% confidence interval was wide: –8% to +36%.

(Peacock *et al.* 2003)

difference, its confidence interval, and its *P* value when that information is already given in tables.

By convention, the results section simply reports the findings and saves comments and interpretation to the discussion section.

4.2.5 Discussion

Many aspects of the discussion will centre on interpreting the findings in the context of previous work and current knowledge. Such discussion may not be intrinsically statistical. However, there are several statistical issues which may require discussion or comment. Box 4.8 lists some of these.

It can be useful to set the sizes of effects and widths of confidence intervals in the context of current knowledge. Box 4.9 gives an example from a study of the adverse health effects of outdoor air pollution.

The study had in general found very similar effect sizes to those previously reported by others. For this particular outcome, the estimate was higher than one reported previously but the current study's 95% confidence interval was wide. Hence findings of the two studies were not inconsistent with each other.

In some studies, many hypothesis tests are performed, increasing the possibility of spurious significant results (type I errors). Where a single and unexpected significant result has been found, it is sensible to view this cautiously and discuss the possibility that it is a false-positive finding. This problem is common in exploratory studies.

Sometimes there are unavoidable limitations in the design or statistical analysis used. This can often happen with student projects where there are tight time constraints, but can happen with other studies. In such cases any limitations and their potential implications should be clearly described and discussed. In practice, no study is perfect and all have some limitations. In a well-designed study, the limitations will be outweighed by the study strengths and the results will be robust.

4.3 Special circumstances

4.3.1 Writing abstracts for conferences

Like abstracts for reports, abstracts for oral and poster conference presentations must stand alone, particularly because conference abstracts are often published in their own right. The specification for these abstracts varies from conference to conference but may be structured and will almost certainly have a word limit.

4.3.2 Short reports and research letters

Some journals allow authors to submit short reports or research letters which typically are 500–1000 words in length with only one table or figure allowed. They do not always fit the usual structure and sections such as introduction and methods can be combined. Because of these constraints it can be difficult to write in this type of format, but it is ideal for a small piece of work.

Chapter summary

Checklist for writing up a research study

Abstract

- Stand-alone document
- Report main outcome with estimates and 95% CI if possible
- Draw valid conclusions

Introduction

- What is the research question?
- What do we know already?
- What are the gaps?
- What does this study add?

Methods

- Describe study design and conduct
- Choice of subjects
- Sample size
- Data collected
- Statistical analysis

Results

- Describe characteristics of the sample
- Describe findings
- Don't just give P values—present estimates and CIs

Discussion

- Summarise findings
- Describe how they fit with existing knowledge
- Discuss any limitations
- Draw conclusions and make suggestions for future research

CHAPTER 5

Introduction to presenting statistical analyses

5.1 Introduction

This chapter shows how to present descriptive statistical analyses. We will describe how to present the results of the recruitment process, and how to describe the characteristics of the study sample. The examples given will be used to draw out general principles of presenting numerical data and we will give general guidelines for presenting numerical data, such as percentages, *P* values, confidence intervals, etc., and for presenting tables and graphs. We will describe how to present different types of data, such as continuous and binary data, and also make recommendations for presentation for different media, such as papers, dissertations and theses, and oral presentations.

5.2 Presenting numerical data

It is important to present numerical data clearly, accurately, and concisely, so that the message that the data contains is communicated. This is not always straightforward, especially when extracting results from computer packages where many details may be given and where results are given to a high level of precision. For example, statistical packages will usually present a mean to many decimal places. However, if the original data are recorded as whole numbers, then it is misleading to present a mean to several decimal places, as it suggests a spuriously high level of accuracy—one decimal place is sufficient. Similarly, percentages should not be given to more than one decimal place if the actual frequencies are also given. Apart from false precision, the other reason for giving fewer decimal places is to help the reader assimilate the information. A table of means or percentages which is presented with several decimal places is hard to absorb.

The other reason for being selective in presentation is that statistical packages often produce detailed output of the statistical procedures used and not all of it needs to be reported. Further, in particular contexts not all of the results may make sense and so the reader has to select carefully which to present. In this book we give many examples of which data to select and present from Stata and SPSS outputs. For example, in Figure 5.5, where arithmetic, geometric, and harmonic means are given by Stata, only the geometric mean is relevant and needed.

The presentation of P values can cause some difficulty. The actual P value should usually be given, whether or not the results are statistically significant. Two significant figures are sufficient. Sometimes packages give very small P values, such as $P = 0.0000$. This does not mean that the P value equals zero but that the calculated P value is smaller than 0.0001 and is therefore 0.0000 to four decimal places. We recommend presenting this as $P < 0.0001$ rather than $P = 0.0000$. Similarly, $P = 1.0000$ does not mean that the P value is exactly 1, but that it is 1.0000 to four decimal places and we recommend presenting this as $P > 0.999$. Box 5.1 gives a summary of guidelines for a range of statistics.

BOX 5.1 **HELPFUL TIPS**

Presenting numerical data and common statistics

Proportions

◆ Give to two significant figures (e.g. 0.25, 0.0056)

◆ Give numbers as well as the actual proportion unless obvious

◆ Use percentage or rate per 1000, 10 000, etc. if proportion is very small

Percentages

◆ Give percentages less than 10 or greater than 90 to one decimal place (e.g. 5.2%, 93.8%)

◆ Consider giving percentages between 10% and 90% as whole numbers, unless the extra precision is needed (e.g. 27% vs 27.3%)

◆ Give numbers as well as actual percentage unless obvious but make clear which is which

◆ Do not use percentages if sample is less than 10

BOX 5.1 *(Continued)*

Mean, SD, SE

◆ Present to one more significant figure than original data

◆ Do not use +/− or ± as this is potentially ambiguous Use 'mean (SD) = . . .' or 'mean (SE) = . . .'

CIs

◆ Present to one more significant figure than original data

◆ Present as '*x* to *y*' or '*x*, *y*' not '*x*–*y*' since this is ambiguous if negative values are possible

P values

◆ Present actual P values wherever possible whether significant or not

◆ Give no more than two significant figures, e.g.
$0.0392 \rightarrow 0.039$
$0.596 \rightarrow 0.60$

◆ If package gives $P = 0.0000$ present as $P < 0.0001$

◆ If package gives $P = 1.0000$ present as $P > 0.999$

* or ** or ***

◆ Not necessary if the actual P value is given

◆ Can be useful where space is limited and CIs are given

◆ Indicate statistical significance at different levels

◆ Usual meaning:
* $P < 0.05$, ** $P < 0.01$, *** $P < 0.001$

Notes

◆ *Significant figures*: these are non-zero digits, e.g. 0.00568 to two significant figures is 0.0057

◆ *Decimal places*: these are the number of digits after the decimal point, e.g. 0.00568 to two decimal places is 0.01. Retain right-hand zeros, e.g. 3.02 to one decimal place is 3.0 not 3

◆ It is usually necessary to select appropriate results from computer output and edit for presentation. All results given may not make sense in a given context

◆ When keeping numbers for further calculation, retain more significant figures than suggested above to maintain accurate calculations (retain all if in doubt)

◆ Rules for rounding 5s:
$0.0325 \rightarrow 0.033$
$0.0324 \rightarrow 0.032$

5.3 Beginning the results section

Before performing the main analyses it is important to describe how the sample was obtained and the main relevant characteristics of that sample. The actual recruitment methodology should be described in the methods section of a paper (see Chapter 4, section 4.2.3) but the numbers of patients actually recruited, response rates, and reasons for non-response should be described at the beginning of the results section. As well as giving the numbers of subjects, it is often useful to describe key characteristics of the group which might affect the results or the generalisability of the results to other patient groups.

5.4 Describing the results of the recruitment process

Box 5.2 gives the key points to consider when describing the results of the recruitment process, from the sampling frame through to the patients included in the analysis. This allows the reader to assess whether the results are likely to be biased in any way and also demonstrates that the study has been carefully carried out and that the results can be trusted.

BOX 5.2 **INFORMATION**

Key points in describing the results of the recruitment process

- Sampling frame

- Number of subjects originally selected

- Number of subjects subsequently excluded because of ineligibility

- Number of non-responders

- Reasons for non-response if known

- Comparison of responders and non-responders if possible

- Number of subjects withdrawing before completing the study

For all randomised trials a flowchart should be included as recommended in the CONSORT guidelines (see Chapter 12). However, a flow chart can be useful for other studies too. In the Wandsworth Heart and Stroke Study, 3606 patients were initially selected from nine general practice lists but only 1577 patients were included in the analysis. Figure 5.1 shows a flowchart illustrating the steps between the sample chosen and that analysed. Many patients had moved away and so would not have been included had the lists been up to date, and hence were removed before

the response rate was calculated. Giving all the figures makes it clear what has happened, and shows that the response rate is probably an underestimate as some of those who did not reply may also have moved away.

5.5 Assessing non-response bias

We have to accept that every person has the right to refuse to take part in medical research but the resulting effects on the results should not be ignored. As much information on non-responders as possible should be obtained to allow potential bias due to non-response to be assessed. Box 5.3 shows that in the Wandsworth Heart and Stroke Study more women than men agreed to take part, possibly because of the difficulty in attending for the research interview during the working day. In addition, some subjects who refused to attend for examination agreed to complete a postal questionnaire. The replies to this questionnaire can be used for further assessment of non-response bias.

BOX 5.3 **EXAMPLE**

Assessing non-response bias
Wandsworth Heart and Stroke Study
Number of patients recruited by sex and ethnic groups ($N = 1577$)

	Males	Females
White	233	290
African origin	208	341
Asian	253	252

- In the sampling frame equal numbers from each sex and ethnic group were selected.

- Table shows an excess of women of African origin

(Cappuccio *et al.* 1997)

5.6 Presenting the results for different media

The way in which the results are presented will depend on whether you are giving a talk, preparing a poster, writing a paper for a scientific journal, or writing a dissertation or thesis.

Reports, dissertations, and theses are usually fairly long and require the results to be presented in detail. Box 5.4 shows an extract from a report of a study into the role of X-rays in the management of low back pain in primary care, and describes the characteristics of the patients recruited.

Wandsworth Heart and Stroke Study

Aim of study: To compare cardiovascular risk factors in three ethnic groups.

Design: Cross-sectional survey with stratified random sampling to obtain equal numbers in each sex/ethnic group category.

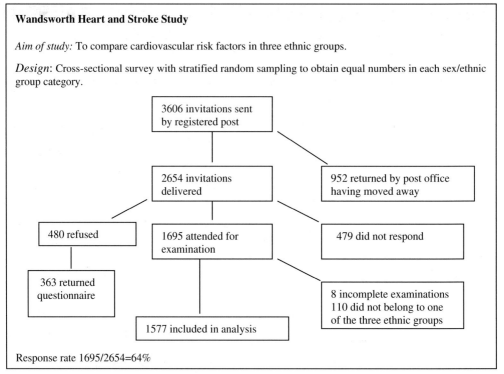

Response rate 1695/2654=64%

Figure 5.1 Flowchart of the recruitment process for the Wandsworth Heart and Stroke Study

BOX 5.4 EXAMPLE

Population profile from a report
Low back pain study
Aim of study To assess the effect of early X-rays for low back pain.

Design Observational study and a randomised controlled trial.

Patient characteristics
The average age of the patients was 41.8 years and 52% were women. Pain had been present for less than one week in 28% of patients and more than 6 months in 22% (table 1). The mean number of consultations in the year before recruitment was 4.0; this compares with a national average of 3.8. The level of pain experienced by these patients is shown in table 2.

Table 1 Length of present episode of back pain

	No. of patients (n = 548)	%
Less than 1 week	156	28
1 week to < 4 weeks	156	28
4 weeks to < 8 weeks	55	10
8 weeks to < 6 months	59	11
6 months and over	122	22

Table 2 Level of pain experienced at recruitment

	No. of patients (n = 555)	%
No pain at all	6	1
Little pain	67	12
Moderate pain	205	37
Quite bad pain	155	28
Very bad pain	101	18
Almost unbearable pain	21	4

(Kerry *et al.* 2000)

BOX 5.5 EXAMPLE

Single concise table from a paper with adjusted and unadjusted estimates

Early Pregnancy Study

Characteristics of 1201 newly pregnant women according to bacterial vaginosis status at recruitment

Characteristics	No. (%) with characteristic	Prevalence (proportion) of women with bacterial vaginosis among		Relative risk (95% CI)	Age-adjusted relative risk (95% CI)
		women with characteristic	women without characteristic		
Age < 25 (n = 1201)	150 (13)	23 (34/150)	13 (140/1051)	1.7 (1.2 to 2.5)**	–
Black Caribbean or Black African (n = 1096)	116 (11)	34 (39/116)	11 (109/980)	3.0 (2.1 to 4.4)***	2.9 (2.0 to 4.2)***
Social class 3 to 5[1] (n = 1036)	415 (40)	16 (68/415)	10 (65/621)	1.6 (1.1 to 2.2)**	1.5 (1.0 to 2.1)*
Single, widowed, or divorced (n = 1095)	94 (9)	29 (27/94)	12 (116/1001)	2.5 (1.6 to 3.8)***	2.3 (1.5 to 3.7)***
Previous contraception oral or none (n = 1084)	682 (63)	15 (101/682)	11 (43/402)	1.4 (0.97 to 2.0)	1.4 (0.97 to 2.0)
No previous pregnancies (n = 1094)	388 (35)	11 (43/388)	15 (107/706)	0.73 (0.51 to 1.0)	0.73 (0.51 to 1.0)
Previous termination of pregnancy (n = 1087)	270 (25)	22 (59/270)	11 (87/817)	2.1 (1.5 to 2.9)***	2.0 (1.5 to 2.8)***

[1] For women who were unemployed or students, partner's social class was used when available.

$* P < 0.05, ** P < 0.01, *** P < 0.001$

Description

Results section

Bacterial vaginosis was more common in younger women, those of African origin, in lower social classes, and those with a history of termination of pregnancy (table).

(Oakeshott *et al*. 2002)

Papers for journals usually have word limits, but need to contain sufficient information for the reader to critically appraise the study. Therefore results need to be presented very concisely, usually in tables and text, rather than in graphs. Box 5.5 shows how a single table can display a great deal of information very concisely. The prevalences of bacterial vaginosis in women with and without each characteristic are shown side by side, so that they can be compared. The most appropriate comparison statistic is the ratio of the prevalences (the relative risk) and this is

shown alongside the relative risk adjusting for age. (This was carried out using the Cox proportional hazards model; see Chapter 11). By setting the unadjusted and adjusted relative risks side by side, the effect of adjustment can easily be seen. In this way, a considerable amount of information can be summarised in one table.

Graphs in papers should only be used when really necessary to convey information that cannot be presented satisfactorily in tables. This is usually when we want to plot the actual data values such as a scattergram (e.g. Box 9.3), or to plot individual study results in a meta-analysis.

The purpose of oral presentations and posters is to convey a key message quickly. Simple tables and graphs are usually more appropriate than complicated tables and solid text. It will often be necessary to omit some of the details from tables that would be presented in a paper. Box 5.6 shows a simplified version of the table in Box 5.5 that would be suitable for a poster or slide. Alternatively, the results could be displayed graphically as in Figure 5.2. The level of pain experienced by patients recruited to the Low Back Pain Study that was presented in a table in Box 5.4, is shown as a graph in Figure 5.3.

When preparing slides for oral presentations care should be taken not to make the font too small and so difficult to read. This in itself will, of course, restrict the amount of information that can be presented. In addition, it may be less distracting for the audience to be presented with small amounts of information at one time, and several simple slides may be better than one complicated one.

Posters need to be attractive and eye-catching; if the poster does not quickly gain the interest of viewers, there is a danger that they will simply walk past. Graphs are a useful way of presenting key findings in a colourful way so that the main message can be understood easily.

Boxes 5.7 and 5.8 give a list of guidelines to consider when deciding how to present data. These

---

BOX 5.6 EXAMPLE

Table suitable for an oral presentation

Table. Relative risk of bacterial vaginosis in 1201 pregnant women

Risk factor	Relative risk of bacterial vaginosis
Age < 25	1.7 (1.2 to 2.5)**
Afro-Caribbean or black African	3.0 (2.1 to 4.4)***
Social class 3 to 5	1.6 (1.1 to 2.2)**
Single, widowed, or divorced	2.5 (1.6 to 3.8)***
No previous pregnancies	0.7 (0.5 to 1.0)
Previous termination of pregnancy	2.1 (1.5 to 2.9)***

***$P<0.001$; **$P<0.01$

BOX 5.7 HELPFUL TIPS

Guidelines for graphs

- Title should explain what the graph is about and what subjects or observations are included
- Give number of subjects or observations
- Label axes, giving units as appropriate
- Refer to graph in the text
- Does the graph show enough information to justify the space it takes?
- For clarity, use two-dimensional rather than three-dimensional graphs
- For a paper: is the graph necessary? Could the data be presented in another way?
- In a slide or poster: will the text be legible?

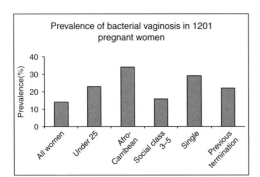

Figure 5.2 Several binary variables on one graph suitable for a poster or talk (example)

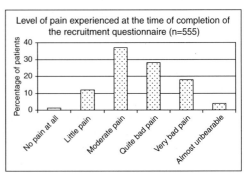

Figure 5.3 Graph for an ordered categorical variable suitable for poster or talk (example)

will help to ensure that the table or graph is clear to the audience. We recommend using two-dimensional graphs rather than three-dimensional graphs, as it is difficult to read numbers and percentages on the latter.

5.7 Drawing up a profile of a group of subjects

Many studies are comparative and hence the presentation of results will focus on the comparison between the groups. However, it is useful to start with a simple description of some of the main features of the sample (e.g. how old they were, the percentage of females), as well as some key variables relevant to the subject of interest. Box 5.4 gives an example taken from a report of a study.

A more concise profile of a group of subjects is given Box 5.9, written for inclusion in a paper. It sets the scene, before the paper continues with a description of the risk factors for bacterial vaginosis (Box 5.5). It describes the age of the women and other factors which may be associated with the prevalence of bacterial vaginosis.

5.8 Drawing graphs

Graphs can be drawn in Stata or SPSS and imported into word-processing or presentation documents (e.g. Word or Powerpoint). Some people use Excel for graphs, as it is commonly available, inputting the summary values from a statistics package. Alternatively, there are specialist graphics packages available.

5.9 Using text to refer to tables and graphs

All tables and graphs should be referred to in the text. It is also helpful to indicate the key findings of the table, as illustrated in Box 5.4. This is more helpful to the reader than 'the results are presented in the table'. The text indicates the message; the data are in the table to support the statement in the text. The same information should not be presented in tables and graphs, and the text should support rather than repeat the tables and graphs.

5.10 Presenting categorical data

5.10.1 Tables for categorical data

Box 5.4 gives an example of a table for an ordered categorical variable, pain experienced. Numbers of subjects in each category are given with the percentages. It is useful to give percentages unless the total number in the sample is very small, say less than 10, when numbers alone will suffice. Giving percentages in this case gives the impression of spurious accuracy. Several variables can be presented in the same table, one underneath the other. This conveys more information concisely together in one table.

Researchers often regroup ordered categories into two categories. This has its drawbacks, particularly if the categories are decided upon after looking at the data, and does lose information. However, it can be useful if conciseness is important. In the Royal College of Radiologists' guidelines concerning X-rays for low back pain, X-rays were not recommended for patients who had been in pain for less than 8 weeks except in certain circumstances. The 'length of episode' variable was therefore grouped into 'less than 8 weeks' and '8 weeks or more' for further analysis. For fuller discussion of grouping data see Kirkwood and Sterne (2003, Chapters 2 and 38).

Where there are only two categories, i.e. binary variables, it is unnecessary to give the numbers in both categories. Instead, only one category need be presented. This makes tables and graphs more concise and easier to absorb. For example, Figure 5.2 simply shows the percentages with bacterial vaginosis, and does not show the percentages without.

5.10.2 Graphs for categorical data

Ordered categories can be presented in a bar chart (Fig. 5.3). Where we wish to compare two groups of subjects, these can be presented as bars in a different colour or shading beside each other (Fig. 5.4). Several binary variables can be presented on one bar chart (Fig. 5.2). The graphs presented here have enough information for one slide of a presentation without containing so much information that it is difficult to absorb quickly.

5.11 Presenting continuous data

5.11.1 Tables and text

Continuous variables are usually summarised by an average, either the mean or the median. A measure of spread of the observations (standard deviation, range, or interquartile range) or a measure of accuracy (standard error or confidence interval) should be given alongside. Box 5.10 gives some tips on which to choose. When quoting standard errors or standard deviations it is important to specify which has been used. The commonly used notation $+/-$ is best avoided and replaced by mean (SD) or

---

BOX 5.10 HELPFUL TIPS

When to present standard deviation, standard error, or confidence interval

Standard deviation

♦ Good descriptor of the distribution of the data values

♦ Use where the variability of the data values is of interest

♦ Use where estimating reference ranges

♦ Can be useful for assessing whether assumptions of the t test hold (see Chapter 7, section 7.2)

♦ Can be difficult to interpret for skewed data

Standard error

♦ Measures precision of an estimate

♦ Related to the confidence interval

♦ Precision is more clearly indicated by the confidence interval, but can use standard error if space limited

♦ Cannot be used where data are transformed and then back-transformed

Confidence interval

♦ Shows the precision of an estimate (e.g. mean, proportion, relative risk etc.)

♦ Generally preferable to standard error (see above)

♦ Can be calculated for geometric means (back-transformed mean of log transformed data)

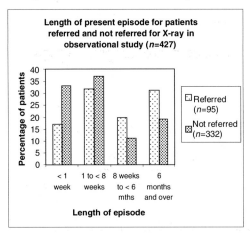

Figure 5.4 Graph comparing two groups of patients suitable for poster or talk (example)

mean (SE). For example 'mean (SD) systolic blood pressure was 121 (19)'. Petrie and Sabin (2000) give a useful list of advantages and disadvantages of the various measures.

When presenting confidence intervals it is preferable to use the word 'to' for separating the two values rather than a dash. A dash is confusing where negative values are possible since it looks the same as a minus sign. Separating the values by a comma is favoured by some journals and is useful if space is limited.

The choice of statistics (e.g. mean or median) should reflect the type of analysis to be carried out. For example, when using a *t* test which compares two means, it is useful to present the means being compared. Analysis of variance and multiple regression are extensions of the *t* test, and therefore it would be consistent to present means for these analyses. A median is the middle rank and hence is more appropriate when rank tests are being used, such as a Mann–Whitney *U* test.

5.11.2 Presenting transformed data

Sometimes the data are highly skewed, but taking the logarithm (often abbreviated to log) of the values produces a distribution which is near Normal. In this case we may wish to do the statistical analysis on the log-transformed data (see sections 7.3.2 and 8.2.2 for examples). However, the log data will be difficult for readers to interpret, and should be back-transformed by anti-logging to return to the original scale. Log-transforming data, calculating a mean, and then back-transforming gives the geometric mean. This is equivalent to taking the *n*th root of the product of all the original observations. Sometimes back-transformation needs to be done by hand on a calculator, while at other times the package may produce the back-transformed results. In Stata, geometric means and their confidence intervals can be calculated directly, as in Figure 5.5, while in SPSS the results need to be back-transformed on a calculator. Figure 5.6 shows how to obtain confidence intervals for a mean in SPSS.

Note that data whose distribution is skewed and which follow a Normal distribution after log transformation are sometimes referred to as following a 'log Normal distribution'.

Other transformations can also be used such as the square root, reciprocal, and angular transforms, and like the log transform these transformations

---

The variable *hdl* is HDL cholesterol and is positively skew. Therefore it was log-transformed to give Normally distributed data. Analysis is on the log transformation of *hdl*, named *loghdl*. The **ci** command can be used to calculate the mean and 95% confidence interval. After analysis the results usually need to be back-transformed on a calculator into the original units. However in Stata the **means** command will calculate the geometric mean which is the same as the anti-log of the mean of the transformed data. The following example shows that these are equivalent. Note that the logs are logs to base e.

```
.gen loghdl=log(hdl)
(108 missing values generated)

. ci loghdl

    Variable |    Obs        Mean    Std. Err.       [95% Conf. Interval]
-------------+-------------------------------------------------------------
      loghdl |    1469     .2734075    .0076731        .258356      .288459
```

log(1.2948) = 0.258356

```
. means hdl

    Variable |    Type       Obs        Mean      [95% Conf. Interval]
-------------+-------------------------------------------------------------
         hdl | Arithmetic    1469     1.372298     1.35127     1.393326
             | Geometric     1469     1.314436      1.2948     1.33437
             | Harmonic      1469     1.258455     1.239012    1.278518
-------------+-------------------------------------------------------------
```

Presentation of results
'The geometric mean (95% confidence interval) of hdl is 1.31(1.29 to 1.33) mmol'.

Figure 5.5 Calculating the confidence interval of a geometric mean in Stata

lcr is the log of serum creatinine concentration and *outcome* denotes whether the patient subsequently died or survived.

While the **Means** command will calculate arithmetic and geometric means it does not provide confidence intervals. To obtain confidence intervals for means use the **Explore** command.
Select 'Analyze'
Select 'Descriptive Statistics'
Select 'Explore'
Move *lcr* to the 'Dependent List'
Move *outcome* to the 'Factor List'. This can be left unfilled for means of the whole sample

The variable analysed here is lcr, i.e. log(creatinine). The values here need to be back-transfomed to obtain the geometric mean exp(4.5787)=97.388

95% confidence interval for geometric mean is given by exp(4.5073) to exp(4.6502) i.e. 90.677 to 104.606

Descriptives

	outcome			Statistic	Std. Error
lcr	alive	Mean		4.5787	.03555
		95% Confidence Interval for Mean	Lower Bound	4.5073	
			Upper Bound	4.6502	
		5% Trimmed Mean		4.5788	
		Median		4.5326	
		Variance		.062	
		Std. Deviation		.24888	
		Minimum		4.03	
		Maximum		5.09	
		Range		1.07	
		Interquartile Range		.35	
		Skewness		.020	.340
		Kurtosis		-.480	.668
	dead	Mean		4.6857	.04840
		95% Confidence Interval for Mean	Lower Bound	4.5889	
			Upper Bound	4.7826	
		5% Trimmed Mean		4.6552	
		Median		4.6151	
		Variance		.143	
		Std. Deviation		.37800	
		Minimum		4.11	
		Maximum		6.08	
		Range		1.97	
		Interquartile Range		.37	
		Skewness		1.430	.306
		Kurtosis		2.989	.604

Presentation of results
'The geometric mean (95% confidence interval) of serum creatinine among survivors is 97(91 to 105) μmol/L and 108 (98 to 119)μmol/L among those who died'.

Figure 5.6 Calculating the confidence interval of a geometric mean in SPSS

also lead to problems in interpreting effect sizes. The choice of transformation depends on the degree of skewness, and the requirement to have an estimate of effect and confidence interval. Further discussion is beyond the scope of this book but more details are given by Bland (2000).

5.11.3 Presenting different types of data in one table

It can be useful to be able to present all variables with a common theme in one table. Box 5.11 shows the cardiovascular risk variables measured in the Wandsworth Heart and Stroke Study and includes continuous variables, untransformed and transformed, and categorical variables. Smoking and diabetes have been included as the percentage smoking and the percentage diabetic. Arithmetic means have been used for blood pressure, but HDL cholesterol was log-transformed for analysis, and so the geometric mean has been presented and indicated by a footnote. Another example of presenting several types of data with a common theme is given in Box 4.7.

5.11.4 Presenting continuous data in graphs

Often we use graphs, such as histograms and Normal plots, to assess the nature of a distribution (whether it is skewed or symmetric) and for assessing outliers (e.g. Fig 2.4). These are useful in the

---

BOX 5.11 EXAMPLE

Presenting several types of variables with a common theme in one table

Table. Age adjusted means (95% confidence interval) of cardiovascular risk variables for men in the Wandsworth Heart and Stroke Study (*n* = 694)

Variable	Mean (95% CI)
Age (years)	50.6 (50.2 to 51.0)
Systolic blood pressure (mm Hg)	131 (129 to 132)
Diastolic blood pressure (mm Hg)	83 (82 to 84)
Total cholesterol (mmol/l)	5.8 (5.7 to 5.9)
HDL cholesterol (mmol/l)[1]	1.18 (1.15 to 1.20)
Current smoking (%)	28 (25 to 31)
Diabetes (%)	14 (11 to 16)

[1] Geometric mean.

Notes

- All results are presented with confidence intervals
- Smoking and diabetes are binary, and expressed as percentages, indicated with a % sign
- HDL cholesterol is log-transformed for analysis; footnote indicates geometric mean

---

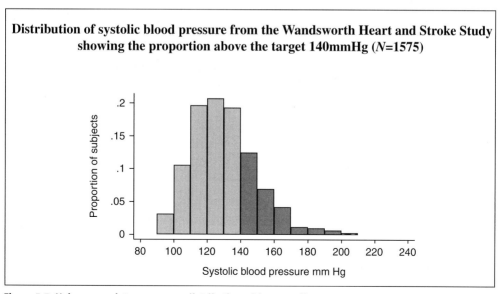

Distribution of systolic blood pressure from the Wandsworth Heart and Stroke Study showing the proportion above the target 140mmHg (*N*=1575)

Figure 5.7 Using a graph to compare a distribution with a cut-off

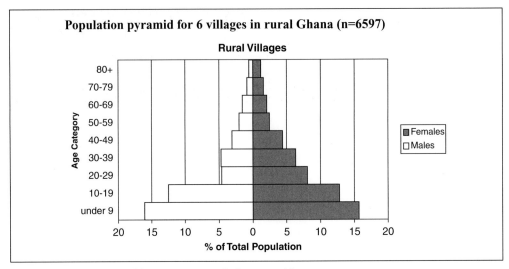

Figure 5.8 Displaying two histograms: a population pyramid

process of verifying assumptions about the data as in sections 7.2 and 8.2, but are not usually presented in a paper because of lack of space. In a dissertation or thesis the graphs might be useful to help explain the methodology; for example, if the data were transformed.

Graphs may be useful if the distribution of a key continuous variable is of interest, for example when calculating a Normal range or comparing the distribution of the data with a predefined cut-off. Figure 5.7 shows the distribution of systolic blood pressure among all subjects in the Wandsworth Heart and Stroke Study, with the cut-off of 140 mmHg indicated by shading the graph. This cut-off is commonly used to define hypertension.

Another situation where the distribution itself rather than the mean is of key interest is in the age–sex profile of a country. These can be shown as a population pyramid which is similar to a histogram but using the vertical axis for age (Fig. 5.8). In the communities studied in rural Ghana (Kerry 2005a) a large proportion of the population were under 20 and there were fewer men in their twenties and thirties than women. This is a rural population and the men may have migrated to work. Population pyramids from African nations now show a lack of men and women in their twenties, thirties and forties because of the AIDS epidemic. Such trends cannot be deduced from the mean and standard deviations alone.

Chapter summary

Presenting statistical analyses

♦ Be careful and selective in presenting numerical data especially when extracting results from computer output

♦ Tables and graphs need to be clear enough to stand alone

♦ Graphs need to convey sufficient information to justify the space they require

♦ Present results concisely in papers, concentrating on tables and text, and only using graphs where information cannot be presented in a table

♦ Use simple tables and graphs for oral presentations and posters

♦ Before doing the main statistical analysis:

*Describe the results of the recruitment process from the selection of subjects through to the analysis
*Draw up a profile of the subjects recruited

CHAPTER 6

Single group studies

6.1 Introduction

Single group studies are often descriptive rather than analytical and aim to produce estimates of quantities such as the prevalence of a condition, or the sensitivity and specificity of a screening test, or a reference range for a measurement. In such studies it is particularly important to describe how the sample was chosen, the characteristics of the sample, and how the outcomes were defined and measured.

For example, the prevalence of hypertension may vary according to how many blood pressure measurements are taken, with a lower prevalence being obtained when three measurements are taken compared with two, since an individual's blood pressure tends to fall with successive measurement. However, if we wish to investigate whether blood pressure is related to body mass index, a systematic bias in the measurement of blood pressure is unlikely to affect the relationship between the two variables. Finally, note that a measure of precision such as a confidence interval should be given as well as the proportions themselves.

In this chapter we will describe how to present prevalence studies and the results of screening studies.

6.2 Prevalence studies

To illustrate presenting prevalence studies, we will use the data from the chlamydia study previously referred to in Chapter 3. The study's aim was to estimate the prevalence of chlamydial infection in women aged 16–34 who were having cervical smear tests in Inner London general practices.

Figure 6.1 shows the Stata output which calculates the proportion of women with the infection and a 95% confidence interval.

There is no straightforward way to calculate a 95% confidence interval for a single proportion in SPSS and so users can either do the calculation using a calculator and the relevant formula (see Altman *et al.* 2000, Chapter 6) or use another statistical programme such as CIPROPORTION, an Excel spreadsheet written by Robert Newcombe and available free from his website (www.cardiff.ac.uk, see Box 2.8). This is illustrated in Figure 6.2.

There are several exact methods for calculating confidence intervals for proportions and the Excel spreadsheet in Figure 6.2 uses a different method to the default in Stata, hence the slight difference in the actual values obtained in Figures 6.1 and 6.2.

6.3 **Presenting the results of prevalence studies**

The prevalence of chlamydial infection (0.029) was small and so was presented as a percentage (2.9%) rather than as a proportion as this avoids having a lot of zeros and makes it easier to read (Box 6.1). Some proportions of interest, such as cause-specific mortality, may be even smaller and therefore are expressed as the number of events per 1000 or even per 100000. For example, perinatal mortality is usually expressed as the number of deaths per 1000 births, and so it is best to choose this format to present the proportion.

BOX 6.1 EXAMPLE

Presenting a prevalence

Chlamydia infection in general practice

Aim of the study To estimate the prevalence of chlamydial infection.

Study design Cross-sectional prevalence study.

Patient population 1382 women aged 16–34 presenting for smear tests in 30 Inner London general practices.

Description

Methods section

The prevalence and extract 95% binomial confidence interval were calculated.

Results section

Forty of the 1382 women tested positive for chlamydial infection (2.9%; 95% confidence interval 2.1% to 3.9%).

(Oakeshott *et al.* 1998)

In addition to presenting the actual prevalence and confidence interval, it is important to describe the recruitment process and the main characteristics of the sample obtained to allow the results to be interpreted in context and to make it clear to which population the results can be generalised (see sections 5.3–5.5).

Note that in the original paper (Oakeshott *et al.* 1998) the large sample Normal approximation was used (proportion ± 1.96 standard errors) to calculate the confidence interval, and this gives a slightly

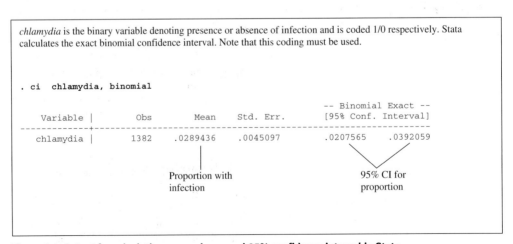

chlamydia is the binary variable denoting presence or absence of infection and is coded 1/0 respectively. Stata calculates the exact binomial confidence interval. Note that this coding must be used.

```
. ci   chlamydia, binomial

                                                    -- Binomial Exact --
        Variable |      Obs         Mean     Std. Err.    [95% Conf. Interval]
    -------------+-------------------------------------------------------------
        chlamydia |     1382     .0289436     .0045097      .0207565     .0392059
```

Proportion with infection

95% CI for proportion

Figure 6.1 Output for calculating a prevalence and 95% confidence interval in Stata

SPSS has been used to obtain the prevalence and numbers of subjects with chlamydia which are then entered into the spreadsheet available on Robert Newcombe's website (Box 2.8, CIPROPORTION).
chlamydia is the binary variable denoting presence or absence of infection and is coded 1/0 respectively.
Select 'Analyze'
Select 'Descriptive Statistics'
Select 'Frequencies'
Move *chlamydia* into the variables box

If there are missing values then the valid percent column should be used. If no missing values, as here, then columns are the same.

chlamydia

		Frequency	Percent	Valid Percent	Cumulative Percent
Valid	No	1342	97.1	97.1	100.0
	Yes	40	2.9	2.9	100.0
	Total	1382	100.0	100.0	

The numbers of subjects are entered into CIPROPORTION below (Box 2.8)

Spreadsheet CIPROPORTION. Confidence intervals for proportions and differences.							
This spreadsheet performs CI calculations for proportions and their differences using good methods.							
To perform these calculations, replace values in **bold** as appropriate.							
Two-sided confidence level required				**95**	%.		
Single proportion. (Wilson EB. J Am Stat Assoc 1927, 22, 209-212).							
Observed	proportion	**40**	out of	**1382**	i.e.	0.0289	
95	% confidence interval		0.0213	to		0.0392	

Figure 6.2 Output for calculating a prevalence in SPSS

different interval. The large sample assumption was reasonable because the numbers were large. However, the large sample Normal method for a single proportion is not routinely available in Stata and so we have used the exact binomial method here.

When the sample is small or there are few subjects with the condition, the exact binomial method must be used to calculate the confidence intervals otherwise invalid values may be obtained. A rule of thumb is that the exact method should be used if the number of subjects both with and without the condition is less than five. If you have a confidence interval for a proportion with a negative lower limit or an upper limit above 1, this is an indication that the large sample assumptions are not met. In such cases the negative limits should not be reset to zero, nor should limits which exceed 1 be reset to 1, since

the confidence limits will then be too narrow. Instead, the exact method should be used.

6.4 **Screening studies: sensitivity and specificity**

These studies are used to evaluate the usefulness of a new screening technique to predict future adverse events. Sensitivity and specificity are calculated to summarise the performance of the new test compared with a 'gold standard' diagnosis.

To illustrate the presentation of sensitivity and specificity, we will use data from a sub-study of the larger UKOS study. The aim of the sub-study was to validate a parental questionnaire as a substitute for a specialist clinical assessment in children who had been born very prematurely. The parental questionnaire measured cognitive development at age 2 years in children who had been born very prematurely by deriving a score from information collected on vocabulary, sentence complexity, and non-verbal cognition. The validation study sought to identify the particular parental questionnaire score that corresponded to a set point on the clinical assessment scale used to identify children with developmental delay. Hence the clinical assessment was regarded as the gold standard and the parental questionnaire as the new screening test.

6.5 Presentation of sensitivity and specificity

Sometimes sensitivity and specificity are given as proportions and sometimes as percentages. It does not really matter since the proportions are usually close to 1 and so there is no confusion as to which have been used. We will use percentages here.

Box 6.2 shows the presentation of the validation study of the screening tool. Figure 6.3 shows how to calculate the sensitivity and specificity in Stata.

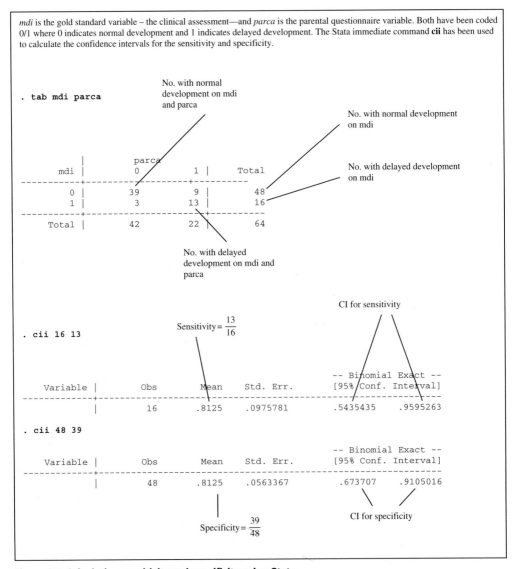

Figure 6.3 **Calculating sensitivity and specificity using Stata**

Note that this was a two-stage process with the numbers obtained from the two-way table being entered manually into the program. The procedure would be similar in SPSS but the spreadsheet would be used as in Figure 6.2.

BOX 6.2 EXAMPLE

Presenting sensitivity and specificity

UKOS validation study

Aim of study To validate a new screening tool for cognitive function in children.

Study design Cross-sectional screening study.

Patient population 64 parents and their children aged 2 years who were born very prematurely.

Description

Methods section

Sensitivity and specificity were calculated with exact 95% binomial confidence intervals.

Results section

Twenty-five percent of children (16/64) scored below the cut-off for normal development using the MDI clinical assessment. Thirteen of the 16 were correctly classified as developmentally delayed by the parental questionnaire giving a sensitivity of 81% (95% CI: 54% to 96%). Of the 48 children classified as having normal development, 39 were correctly classified by the parental questionnaire giving a specificity of 81% (95%CI: 67% to 91%).

(Johnson *et al.* 2004)

Hand calculation using the large sample approximation may be dubious because sensitivity and specificity are likely be close to 100% and so the approximations involved may not be reasonable.

6.6 Comment on results

Figure 6.3 shows that the sensitivity and specificity in the validation study were fairly high, indicating that the parental questionnaire performed reasonably well. However, the confidence intervals were wide, especially for the sensitivity, which was based on only 16 observations.

6.7 Screening studies for rare conditions

It is important to give the actual numbers when presenting sensitivity and specificity. In addition, a confidence interval is usually informative. These

---

BOX 6.3 EXAMPLE

Screening study with rare condition

Ultrasound study

Study aim

To investigate the use of Doppler ultrasound in pregnancy at 23 weeks gestation to predict the development of adverse perinatal outcomes in twin pregnancies.

Study population

360 pregnant women carrying twins, who had had Doppler ultrasound examination at 22–24 weeks gestation.

Ultrasound measurements

Pulsatility index ($\geq 95^{th}$ centile)
Bilateral notches

Outcomes

Pre-eclampsia
Fetal growth retardation (FGR)
Abruption
Intrauterine death
Preterm delivery ≤ 32 weeks

Extract of results

Sensitivity (95% CI) for pulsatility index ($\geq 95^{th}$ centile):

Pre-eclampsia	7/21=33% (15%, 57%)
FGR in both twins	3/31=10% (2%, 26%)
Abruption	2/3=67% (9%, 99%)
Intrauterine death	2/6=33% (4%, 78%)
Delivery ≤ 32 wk	8/43=19% (8%, 33%)

Comment

Two screening measures were tested on several outcomes. Adverse outcomes were rare so sensitivities were all based on small numbers even though the total sample size, 360, was quite large. Thus the confidence intervals were very wide showing that the estimates were imprecise.

(Yu *et al.* 2002)

allow the reader to judge the precision of the estimates and are especially important when there are very few 'positives' and therefore the precision of the sensitivity is low.

Box 6.3 shows an example of a screening study where the total number of subjects studied was large (360), but the number who were positive for various outcomes was much smaller (ranging from 3 to 43) because the outcomes were rare. Thus, despite the large overall sample size, the estimates of sensitivity were based on small numbers and were imprecise. This situation is not uncommon and is another reason why it is important to include the numbers from which sensitivity and specificity were calculated, and the confidence intervals, as well as the proportions themselves.

are several possible values. This method was used in the UKOS validation study described earlier. Details of ROC curves are omitted here but a general description can be found in Altman *et al.* (1994).

Sometimes it is useful to calculate other statistics such as the positive predictive value and the negative predictive value. The presentation of these statistics is the same as for sensitivity and specificity as they are also essentially simple proportions.

It is possible to compare the performance of two or more screening tools by comparing quantities like the sensitivity and specificity, and the area under the ROC curve. Such analyses take account of the precision of the estimates. Details are beyond the scope of this book.

6.8 Extensions to sensitivity and specificity

Receiver operating characteristic (ROC) curves can be used to determine the best cut-off when there

6.9 Further reading

The references given in Box 6.4 are those that we have found particularly useful for the specific topics listed.

BOX 6.4 INFORMATION

Further references to statistical details presented in this chapter

Confidence intervals for single proportions

Altman (1991, Chapter 10), Altman *et al.* (2000, Chapter 6), Armitage *et al.* (2002, Chapter 4), Bland (2000, Chapter 8), Campbell and Machin (1999, Chapter 5), Kirkwood and Sterne (2003, Chapter 15), Petrie and Sabin (2000, Chapter 23)

Sensitivity and specificity

Altman (1991, Chapter 14), Armitage *et al.* (2002, Chapter 19), Bland (2000, Chapter 15), Kirkwood and Sterne (2003, Chapter 36), Petrie and Sabin (2000, Chapter 35)

Chapter summary

Presenting single proportions

- Give numbers of subjects as well as the proportion or percentage

- Choose an appropriate presentation for a prevalence which avoids too many zeros (e.g. percentage, rate per 1000, rate per 100000 etc.)

- Sensitivity and specificity can be presented either as proportions or as percentages as the values tend to be close to 100%

- Present 95% confidence intervals for prevalence/sensitivity/specificity unless the number of subjects is very small

Comparing two groups

7.1 Introduction

Subjects are often grouped together according to some characteristic and then the groups are compared. The groups might be different treatment groups in a clinical trial, subjects with different exposures to a risk factor, or cases and controls in an unmatched case–control study. In a case–control study, if the cases and controls are matched together so that each case has one or more controls matched to it, methods for analysing matched data should be used as described in Chapter 8. In this chapter we will consider three different situations: comparing two groups using a *t* test, comparing two groups using a Mann–Whitney *U* test, and comparing two proportions. Chapter 11 describes how to compare survival curves in two or more groups.

7.2 Graphical presentation of continuous unpaired data

In many situations it will be sufficient to describe the data using summary statistics such as the mean and standard deviation, or the median and range. Sometimes the distribution is of interest and a graphical presentation which allows the two groups to be compared is useful. This will be illustrated by two examples from the same study. Twelve villages in Ghana took part in a health education trial to reduce salt intake (Kerry *et al.* 2005a). Blood pressure and body mass index were measured before the intervention began. We present the body mass index for 338 women living in six semi-urban villages compared with 290 women living in six rural villages. Figure 7.1 shows the two histograms on the same axes. This is easier to compare than two completely separate histograms. The figure shows that body mass index is higher in the semi-urban women, with a long tail at the

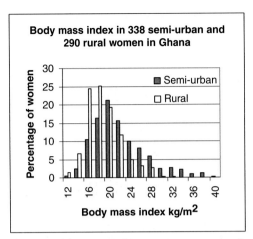

Figure 7.1 Histograms of two groups on one graph

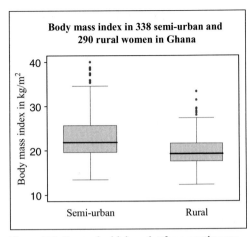

Figure 7.2 Box and whisker plot for a continuous variable in two groups

upper end of the distribution. Body mass index is still skew in the rural areas but less so, and a greater proportion of rural women are underweight (as defined by a body mass index below 18 kg/m^2).

Alternatively, a box and whisker plot can be drawn as shown in Figure 7.2. The thick black lines across the boxes represent the median of each group. The top and bottom of each box indicates the upper and lower quartiles and so the box length is the interquartile range (IQR). Extreme values or outliers are indicated as separate points. In this figure extreme values are only seen at the top end of the distribution as it is positively skewed and all the observations at the lower end fall within the 'expected' range. In Stata and SPSS, outliers are defined as observations which are more extreme than 1.5 × IQR from either quartile. The box plot shows similar features to the histogram in Figure 7.1 and it is a matter of personal choice which type of graph one uses.

The numbers of women in these samples were large, leading to fairly smooth histograms. With small datasets, where a histogram may be uneven, a scatterplot of the data may be more useful. To illustrate this we will use the percentage of villagers who had electricity in their homes in each of the twelve villages. This is shown in Figure 7.3 (Kerry *et al.* 2005a).

There were six villages in each group. Two rural villages had no electricity at all. So that two points can be seen, the points have been 'jittered'. This is a technique which adds a small amount of random variability to the placing of the points so that all points can be seen. The graph shows that in semi-urban villages around 80% of the respondents had electricity and there was little variability between the

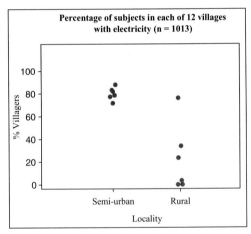

Figure 7.3 Scatterplot for a continuous variable comparing two groups

villages. On the other hand, in rural villages there were far fewer homes with electricity but a much greater difference between villages.

7.2.1 Graphical presentation of more than two groups

The box and whisker plot and the scatterplot can easily be extended to more than two groups. In Figure 7.2, body mass index for men in semi-urban and rural areas could also be shown on the same axes.

7.3 Continuous unpaired data: the two-sample *t* test

A total of 110 patients with peripheral vascular disease were recruited to a cohort study to investigate the predictors of mortality (Missouris *et al.* 2004). The analysis uses a *t* test to compare the mean blood pressure at recruitment in those who subsequently died with those who survived. Before carrying out a *t* test we must check that the assumptions of the *t* test hold (see Box 7.1).

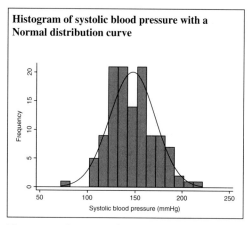

Figure 7.4 Histogram of a variable to check for Normality

BOX 7.1 INFORMATION

The two-sample *t* test

The *t* test is a test of significance which gives an estimate of difference and a confidence interval as well as a *P* value

Null hypothesis Difference between the two population means is zero.

Most suitable for continuous variables but can also be used for scores.

Assumptions Data are Normally distributed and standard deviations of the two groups are the same.

Deviations from the assumptions The *t* test can be used when:

◆ Data are symmetric even if non-Normal

◆ Data are symmetric but display digit preference

◆ Two samples are the same size even if data are moderately skewed

◆ Data are highly skewed but the groups are large (>50 in each group)

Checking the assumptions

◆ Does a histogram of the data look symmetric? Note that small samples will often display an uneven distribution which can be ignored

◆ Are the SDs similar? If the SD is larger in the group with the largest mean this may indicate skewness

◆ If data are skew, try to transform; otherwise power is lost

Unequal variances

◆ Often an indication of skewness

◆ Consider using modified *t* test such as Satterthwaite's test, available in both Stata and SPSS

Levene's test for equality of variance

◆ Routinely given by SPSS but it is of limited value

◆ When samples are small, the test may not pick up important differences

◆ When samples are large, the test may pick up differences which will not affect the results of the test

---

If the assumptions do not hold, then we may fail to detect a real difference or have confidence intervals which are too wide. The histogram (Figure 7.4) shows that systolic blood pressure is very slightly skew but not enough to invalidate the *t* test. For a full discussion of the *t* test and its assumptions, see Bland (2000, Chapter 10). If the assumptions do not hold, then a transformation might be considered (section 7.3.2) or a Mann–Whitney *U* rank test might be used (section 7.4).

7.3.1 Presenting the results of a *t* test

Since the *t* test tests the hypothesis that two population means are the same, the sample mean and the standard deviation are the most appropriate descriptive statistics to report along with the difference in means and its 95% confidence interval. The use of the standard deviation rather than the standard error for the two groups allows the assumptions of equal standard deviation to be assessed by the reader. Showing the means of the two groups helps to describe the patient groups and is also a check on the direction of the difference in means.

The results of the two-sample *t* test using Stata and SPSS are shown in Figures 7.5 and 7.6, and an illustration of how to present these findings is given in Box 7.2. The analysis shows that those who died had 4 mmHg higher mean systolic and diastolic blood pressure at recruitment than those who survived, but the difference is not significant.

BOX 7.2 EXAMPLE

Presenting the results of a *t* test

Peripheral vascular disease study

Aim of study To assess the long-term survival of patients with peripheral vascular disease (PVD) and to investigate the impact of the presence of risk factors on mortality.

Study design Cohort study.

Patient population Consecutive patients with PVD and intermittent claudication who were referred for angiography and found to have angiographic evidence of PVD.

Aim of analysis To compare baseline blood pressure in survivors and those who died.

Table. Comparison of blood pressure in survivors and those who died.

	Mean (SD)		Difference	
	Died (N = 61)	**Survived (N = 49)**	**(95% CI)**	**P value**
Systolic blood pressure (mmHg)	149 (26)	145 (21)	4 (−5 to 13)	0.37
Diastolic blood pressure (mmHg)	78 (14)	74 (10)	4 (−1 to 9)	0.085

Description

Methods section

Mean blood pressure values between patients who died and who survived were compared using unpaired *t* tests.

Results section

Mean blood pressure values were 4 mmHg higher in those who died than in those who survived, but this difference was not statistically significant (table).

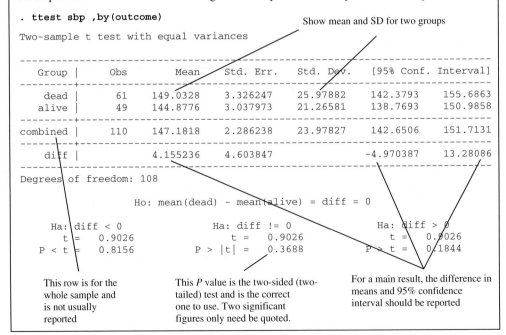

The variable *sbp* is systolic blood pressure and *outcome* is self-explanatory.
The information given by the *t* test procedure is very comprehensive and items need to be selected from the output. All means and error terms are given to many more decimal places than is required.

```
. ttest sbp ,by(outcome)                    Show mean and SD for two groups

Two-sample t test with equal variances

-----------------------------------------------------------------------------
   Group |     Obs        Mean    Std. Err.   Std. Dev.   [95% Conf. Interval]
---------+-------------------------------------------------------------------
    dead |      61    149.0328    3.326247    25.97882    142.3793    155.6863
   alive |      49    144.8776    3.037973    21.26581    138.7693    150.9858
---------+-------------------------------------------------------------------
combined |     110    147.1818    2.286238    23.97827    142.6506    151.7131
---------+-------------------------------------------------------------------
    diff |             4.155236    4.603847               -4.970387    13.28086
-----------------------------------------------------------------------------
Degrees of freedom: 108

              Ho: mean(dead) - mean(alive) = diff = 0

    Ha: diff < 0                 Ha: diff != 0                 Ha: diff > 0
      t =   0.9026                 t =   0.9026                  t =   0.9026
  P < t =   0.8156            P > |t| =   0.3688              P > t =   0.1844
```

This row is for the whole sample and is not usually reported

This *P* value is the two-sided (two-tailed) test and is the correct one to use. Two significant figures only need to be quoted.

For a main result, the difference in means and 95% confidence interval should be reported

Figure 7.5 Output for an unpaired *t* test in Stata

Select 'Analyze'
Select 'Compare means'
Select 'Independent-Samples T Test'
Move *sbp* into 'Test variable' box
Move *outcome* into 'Grouping variable' box and select (0 v 1) for codes to be compared
The grouping variable must have a numeric coding; here the numeric codes 0 and 1 have been labelled 'alive' and 'dead'
The information here is very comprehensive and items need to be selected from the output. All means and error terms are given to many more decimal places than required.

Show mean and SD
for two groups

Group Statistics

	outcome	N	Mean	Std. Deviation	Std. Error Mean
sbp	alive	49	144.88	21.266	3.038
	dead	61	149.03	25.979	3.326

Independent Samples Test

		Levene's Test for Equality of Variances	
		F	Sig.
sbp	Equal variances assumed	.249	.619
	Equal variances not assumed		

Table continued on next row but appears in SPSS as one table

See Box 7.1 for interpretation of this test. This is not the *P* value for the *t* test

		t-test for Equality of Means					95% Confidence Interval of the Difference	
		t	df	Sig. (2-tailed)	Mean Difference	Std. Error Difference	Lower	Upper
sbp	Equal variances assumed	-.903	108	.369	-4.155	4.604	-13.281	4.970
	Equal variances not assumed	-.922	107.953	.358	-4.155	4.505	-13.085	4.774

P value for the *t* test.
Two significant figures
only need be quoted

For a main result the difference between the means and 95%confidence interval would be reported.Use the upper line.

Figure 7.6 Output for an unpaired *t* test in SPSS

7.3.2 **Logarithmic transformations**

Figure 7.7 shows histograms for a skewed variable, serum creatinine level, before and after log transformation. The data are still slightly skewed after log transformation, but since the groups are fairly equal in size and both are fairly large, the slight skew should not affect the *t* test (see Bland (2000, Chapter 10) for a fuller discussion). The results of these descriptive analyses would not normally be reported in the main body of a report, particularly if space is limited (as in a journal paper), unless the distribution of the variable was of prime interest.

It is worth noting that transforming the data using logarithms will not be suitable for all skewed data and that transformation changes the hypothesis being tested (Box 7.3).

The results of the *t* test using Stata and SPSS are shown in Figures 7.8 and 7.9. Back-transformation with a calculator is required to obtain the ratio of the geometric means and 95% confidence intervals. Since only the 95% confidence intervals can be back-transformed to give sensible results, we suggest that 95% confidence intervals are used throughout as in Box 7.4.

BOX 7.3 INFORMATION

The *t* test on log-transformed data

Null hypothesis The ratio of the population geometric means equals 1.

Used for continuous variables with a positive skew and positive values.

Assumptions Apply to log transformed data: transformed data are Normally distributed and standard deviations of the two groups are the same.

Not suitable for:

- ◆ Highly skewed data as log transformation will not give Normal distribution (e.g. assay results where many subjects have undetectable levels)
- ◆ Cost data where the main interest is usually in the arithmetic mean which relates directly to cost per patient.

Note

- ◆ Data with a small number of zero values can be log-transformed by adding a small constant to the zero values before transformation. If there are many zeros, the data will be highly skewed and this transformation will not work. For other options in such cases see Bland (2000, Chapter 10)

- ◆ Bootstrapping methods can be used to overcome problems with skewed cost data

---

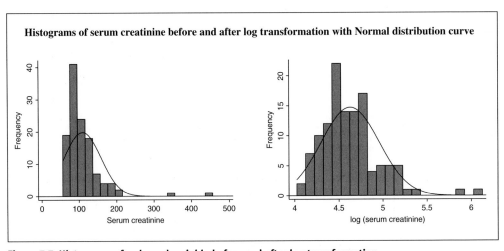

Histograms of serum creatinine before and after log transformation with Normal distribution curve

Figure 7.7 Histograms of a skewed variable before and after log transformation

lcr is the variable for the log transform of creatinine. Do not back-transform standard errors or standard deviations. Commands are the same as in Figure 7.6 but *sbp* has been replace by *lcr*

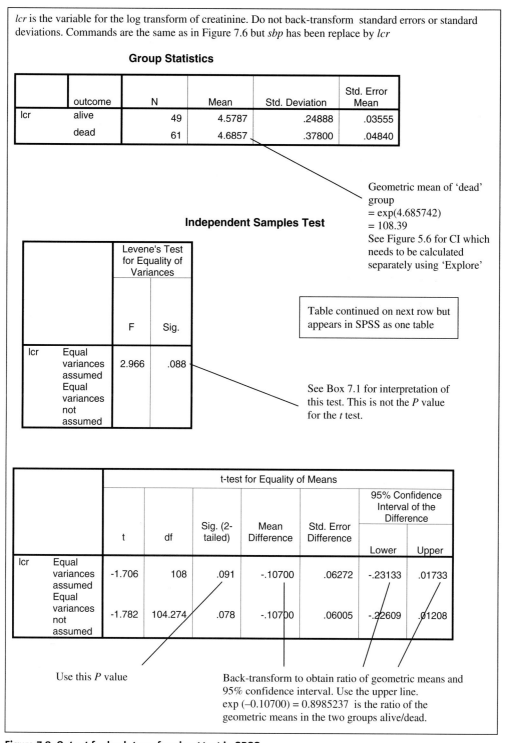

Group Statistics

	outcome	N	Mean	Std. Deviation	Std. Error Mean
lcr	alive	49	4.5787	.24888	.03555
	dead	61	4.6857	.37800	.04840

Geometric mean of 'dead' group
= exp(4.685742)
= 108.39
See Figure 5.6 for CI which needs to be calculated separately using 'Explore'

Independent Samples Test

		Levene's Test for Equality of Variances	
		F	Sig.
lcr	Equal variances assumed	2.966	.088
	Equal variances not assumed		

Table continued on next row but appears in SPSS as one table

See Box 7.1 for interpretation of this test. This is not the *P* value for the *t* test.

		t-test for Equality of Means					95% Confidence Interval of the Difference	
		t	df	Sig. (2-tailed)	Mean Difference	Std. Error Difference	Lower	Upper
lcr	Equal variances assumed	-1.706	108	.091	-.10700	.06272	-.23133	.01733
	Equal variances not assumed	-1.782	104.274	.078	-.10700	.06005	-.22609	.01208

Use this *P* value

Back-transform to obtain ratio of geometric means and 95% confidence interval. Use the upper line.
exp (–0.10700) = 0.8985237 is the ratio of the geometric means in the two groups alive/dead.

Figure 7.8 Output for back-transforming *t* test in SPSS

lcr is the variable for the log transform of creatinine (cr). Do not back-transform standard errors or standard deviations

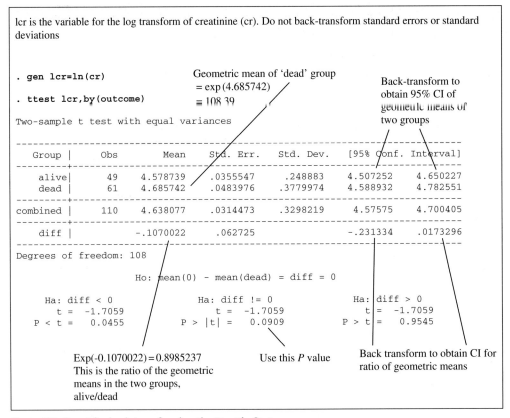

Figure 7.9 Ouput for back-transforming the *t* test in Stata

7.3.3 **Further analysis of the data**

Sometimes we may wish to investigate whether the differences between the means (or the lack of difference) is due to some third factor. One way of doing this is to use multiple regression analysis. Mathematically, multiple regression analysis is an extension of the *t* test and has similar assumptions. If we use multiple regression analysis we can then present the difference in means and the difference in means adjusted for the third factor alongside each other. We show how to perform and present these analyses in Chapter 10.

BOX 7.4 EXAMPLE

Presenting the findings of a t test on log- transformed data

Peripheral vascular disease study

Aim of study To assess the long-term survival of patients with peripheral vascular disease (PVD) and to investigate the impact of the presence of risk factors on mortality.

Study design Cohort study.

Patient population Consecutive patients with PVD and intermittent claudication who were referred for angiography and found to have angiographic evidence of PVD.

Aim of analysis To compare baseline serum creatinine in survivors and those who died.

Table. Comparison of serum creatinine in survivors and those who died

	Geometric mean (95% CI)		Ratio of geometric means (95% CI)	P value
	Survived (N = 49)	Died (N = 61)		
Serum creatinine at baseline (mmol/l)	97 (91, 105)	108 (98,119)	0.90 (0.79,1.02)	0.091

Description

Methods section

Serum creatinine values were positively skew and so the raw data were log-transformed prior to using the t test. The results are presented as geometric means and the ratio of geometric means with 95% confidence intervals.

Results section

Mean serum creatinine values were 10% lower in those who than in those who died, but this difference was not statistically significant (table).

7.4 Mann–Whitney U test

The Mann–Whitney U test is a test based on ranks (equivalent to the Wilcoxon two sample test) for comparing two independent groups. It can be used where there is no suitable Normalizing transformation or the data are in the form of a score (Box 7.5). This test will be illustrated by comparing the number of portions of fruit and vegetables eaten per day by smokers and non-smokers. The data come from the baseline questionnaire of subjects enrolled into a trial of an intervention to increase the consumption of fruit and vegetables among low-income families (Steptoe *et al.* 2003). The data are tabulated in Figure 7.10.

As the Mann–Whitney U test is based on ranks, the median (middle rank) and interquartile range are the most appropriate summary statistics to report; however, the test does not provide a 95% confidence interval, but only a P value.

Figures 7.10 and 7.11 show the output from Stata and SPSS for the fruit and vegetable data, and Box 7.6 shows how this could be presented. Median and interquartile range have been used to present the fruit and vegetable consumption in the two groups.

In situations where there are a small number of possible values and lots of equal values (ties) in the data, the medians may be the same even if there is a tendency for one group to have higher values than the other group. In this case it may be more informative to give the percentage below a cut off point. In the fruit and vegetable consumption study, 69% of non smokers and 90% of smokers consumed less than 5 portions of fruit and vegetables per day. Public health campaigns have promoted eating 5 portions per day so this would seem a good cut off point to use if additional summary data were needed.

smokeas is coded 0 for non-smokers and 1 for smokers. *frandveg* is the number of portions of fruit and vegetables eaten per day.

```
tab frandveg smokeas
```

	SMOKEAS		
FRANDVEG	0	1	Total
0	0	1	1
.5	1	0	1
1	7	7	14
1.5	5	1	6
2	33	21	54
2.5	12	4	16
3	28	26	54
3.5	4	3	7
4	26	19	45
4.5	8	0	8
5	18	3	21
5.5	3	0	3
6	16	3	19
7	9	2	11
7.5	1	0	1
8	5	0	5
9	1	1	2
10	1	0	1
11	1	0	1
13	1	0	1
Total	180	91	271

Figure 7.10a Table for data prior to using Mann–Whitney *U* test from Stata

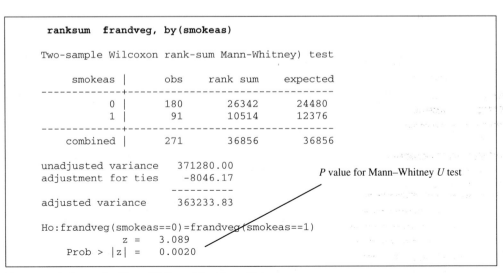

Figure 7.10b Output for Mann–Whitney *U* test from Stata

smokeas is coded 0 for non-smokers and 1 for smokers. *frandveg* is the number of portions of fruit and vegetables eaten per day. The only information from this output which needs to be reported is the *P* value.

Select 'Analyze'

Select 'Non parametric Tests'

Select 'Two Independent-Samples Tests'

Move *frandveg* to 'Test variable' box

Move *smokeas* to the 'Grouping variable' box and enter groups required to compare (*smokeas* comparing 0 v 1)

The 'grouping variable' must have a numeric coding

Ranks

	smokeas	N	Mean Rank	Sum of Ranks
frandveg	0	180	146.34	26342.00
	1	91	115.54	10514.00
	Total	271		

Test Statistics(a)

	frandveg
Mann-Whitney U	6328.000
Wilcoxon W	10514.000
Z	-3.089
Asymp. Sig. (2-tailed)	.002

a Grouping Variable: smokeas

P value for Mann–Whitney *U* test

Figure 7.11 Output for Mann–Whitney *U* test from SPSS

BOX 7.6 EXAMPLE

Presenting the results of a Mann–Whitney *U* test

Eat for life study

Aim of the study To see if a behavioural intervention can increase fruit and vegetable consumption in low-income families.

Study design Randomised controlled trial.

Patient population Patients recruited from one general practice age–sex register.

Aim of analysis To compare fruit and vegetable consumption in smokers and non-smokers.

Description

Methods section

The fruit and vegetable scores from smokers and non-smokers were compared using a Mann–Whitney *U* test. The data are presented as medians and interquartile range (IQR).

Results section

The median (IQR) number of portions of fruit and vegetable eaten per day at baseline among smokers was 3 (2, 4) and 3.75 (2, 5) among non-smokers. Smokers reported significantly lower consumption than non-smokers ($P = 0.002$).

(Steptoe *et al.* 2003)

7.5 Comparing two proportions

7.5.1 The chi-squared test

The simplest test of two proportions is the chi-squared test, often written χ^2. The main uses and assumptions of the test are given in Box 7.7.

The chi-squared test is often used for analysing surveys where the response to various questions is cross-classified by other variables. For example, a student questionnaire on obesity investigated nutrition and exercise in the students' families and friends (Box 7.8). This questionnaire was produced by the students in class, and each student collected data from two friends or family members, thus giving a reasonable total sample size when all data were pooled. (The survey was used as a teaching tool, and therefore is not perfect! However, the

> **BOX 7.7 INFORMATION**
>
> ### The chi-squared test for two proportions
>
> *Null hypothesis* The proportion of individuals in the population with the characteristic is the same in the two groups.
>
> *Suitable for* variables where subjects fall into one of two categories.
>
> *Assumptions* Large sample test. All expected values must be greater than 5.
>
> *Limitations* Significance test only; consider using risk difference, relative risk, or odds ratio to assess the size of the difference between the groups.

BOX 7.8 EXAMPLE

Presenting the results of survey data with several chi-squared tests

Obesity Study

Aim of the study To investigate nutrition, exercise, and attitudes to obesity.

Participants Family and friends of students.

Aim of the analysis To see if reported nutrition, exercise, and attitudes to obesity differed in men and women.

Description

Methods section

The differences in the proportions of men and women responding positively to each question were tested using the chi-squared test. Results are presented as percentages and the corresponding *P* value.

Results section

Table Nutrition, exercise and attitudes to obesity in men and women

Question	Men (N=34)	Women (N=47)	P value
Eats a healthy diet	79% (27/34)	77% (36/47)	0.76
Eats fatty food weekly or more	29% (10/34)	36% (17/47)	0.52
Eats vegetables daily	65% (22/34)	66% (31/47)	0.91
Takes some exercise	71% (24/34)	64% (30/47)	0.52
Thinks obesity is person's own business	64% (21/33)	42% (19/45)	0.062
Thinks obesity is a medical issue for the NHS	27% (9/33)	49% (22/45)	0.054

Eighty-one questionnaires were returned, 34 from men and 47 from women. Most respondents reported eating a healthy diet and the majority eat vegetables every day, eat fatty foods infrequently, and take some exercise. The percentages were similar in men and women. More men than women thought that obesity was a personal affair, and more women than men thought that obesity was an issue for the NHS to deal with. The differences between men and women in these attitude questions were of borderline significance (table).

data are useful for illustrating the presentation of a simple survey.)

7.5.2 Presenting chi-squared tests

When presenting the results of chi-squared tests, new researchers sometimes present each test as a separate table and therefore include unnecessary information given by computer programs. This makes it hard to absorb the findings, and also makes the results section very long. In Box 7.8 we show how several chi-squared tests can be presented concisely in one table. Note that it is unnecessary to give the proportion who respond negatively to the questions as well as the proportions who respond positively where the outcome is dichotomous, since one can easily be deduced from the other. For example, we do not need to give the proportion who take no exercise as well as the proportion who take exercise.

We have not reported the actual chi-square test statistic since we do not think it necessary if the data are given. We have not calculated confidence intervals since the survey was purely descriptive and confidence intervals would not provide any useful additional information. Later on in this chapter we give examples where estimates and confidence intervals should be included. Examples given shortly in this chapter show how to extract the relevant information from Stata and SPSS output for the chi-squared test (Figs 7.12 and 7.13).

Note that the 2×2 chi-squared test is a large sample test and will be invalid in small samples. A rule of thumb that is widely used to define a large sample is one in which all the chi-squared test expected values are greater than 5. The chi-squared test with the continuity correction is better than the ordinary chi-squared test in small sample situations or, alternatively, Fisher's exact test can be used. Fisher's exact test can always be used on 2×2 tables and although it may be slow to compute on less powerful computers, this is rarely a problem nowadays. In a large sample, both Fisher's exact test and the chi-squared test will give similar P values and should therefore lead to the same conclusion.

7.5.3 The chi-squared test and estimates of effect

The main drawback of the chi-squared test is that it is a test of significance only; it does not tell us

---

BOX 7.9 HELPFUL TIPS

Which estimate to use for comparing proportions?

We will call the two proportions p_1 and p_2.

Risk difference: p_1-p_2

- Most straightforward estimate and useful for surveys
- Use if actual size of difference is of interest
- Can be useful for randomised trials as relates to the numbers needed to treat (1/risk difference)

Relative risk: p_1/p_2

- Use if the relative difference is of interest
- Useful when comparing the size of effect for several factors
- Easier to interpret than the odds ratio
- Adjust for other factors using Poisson regression, but this can be problematic when outcome is common
- Do not use for case–control studies

Odds ratio; ad/bc where a, b, c, d are frequencies in 2×2 table

- Approximates to relative risk if outcome is rare
- Can be misinterpreted where outcome is common
- Use for case–control studies
- Easier to adjust for other factors than relative risks
- Adjust for other factors using logistic regression

---

how large the difference between the groups is. There are three main ways to compare proportions: to calculate the difference in the proportions, to calculate the ratio of the proportions, and to calculate the ratio of the odds. These are summarised in Box 7.9. The choice of whether to use a difference or a ratio of proportions depends partly on the context and partly on personal preference.

bv is the binary variable denoting bacterial vaginosis.

tab is useful as it keeps the value labels instead of using 'exposed' and 'unexposed' and 'cases' and 'controls' (non-cases). However, **cs** provides not only the risk of bv in each group but also the relative risk and the risk difference and their 95% confidence intervals. Usually either relative risk or risk difference is reported. For **cs** to give correct relative risk, variables must be coded as 0/1 where 0 = absence of risk factor, 1 = presence of risk factor; 0 = control and 1 = case.

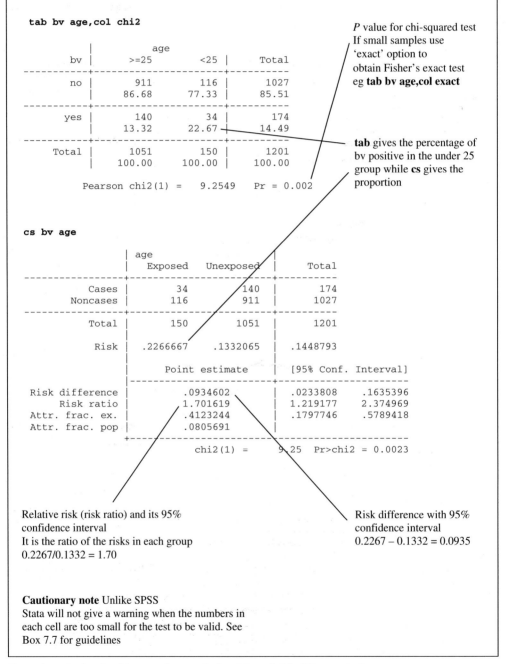

```
tab bv age,col chi2

           |          age
        bv |      >=25        <25 |     Total
-----------+--------------------+----------
        no |       911        116 |      1027
           |     86.68      77.33 |     85.51
-----------+--------------------+----------
       yes |       140         34 |       174
           |     13.32      22.67 |     14.49
-----------+--------------------+----------
     Total |      1051        150 |      1201
           |    100.00     100.00 |    100.00

        Pearson chi2(1) =    9.2549   Pr = 0.002
```

P value for chi-squared test
If small samples use
'exact' option to
obtain Fisher's exact test
eg **tab bv age,col exact**

tab gives the percentage of
bv positive in the under 25
group while **cs** gives the
proportion

```
cs bv age

              |        age
              |   Exposed   Unexposed |     Total
--------------+---------------------+----------
        Cases |        34        140 |       174
     Noncases |       116        911 |      1027
--------------+---------------------+----------
        Total |       150       1051 |      1201
              |
         Risk |  .2266667   .1332065 |  .1448793

              |     Point estimate   | [95% Conf. Interval]
              |---------------------+----------------------
Risk difference |       .0934602     |  .0233808    .1635396
    Risk ratio |       1.701619     |  1.219177    2.374969
 Attr. frac. ex. |     .4123244     |  .1797746    .5789418
 Attr. frac. pop |     .0805691     |
              +---------------------+----------------------
                  chi2(1) =    9.25  Pr>chi2 = 0.0023
```

Relative risk (risk ratio) and its 95%
confidence interval
It is the ratio of the risks in each group
0.2267/0.1332 = 1.70

Risk difference with 95%
confidence interval
0.2267 – 0.1332 = 0.0935

Cautionary note Unlike SPSS
Stata will not give a warning when the numbers in
each cell are too small for the test to be valid. See
Box 7.7 for guidelines

Figure 7.12 Output for chi-squared test, relative risk, and risk difference in Stata

Select 'Analyze'
Select 'Descriptive statistics'
Select 'Crosstabs'
Select row and column variables. To obtain the correct relative risk the risk factor must be the column variable.
Select 'Statistics' and tick boxes for 'Chisq' and 'risk' and row percentages
Risk factor variable was coded 1/2 where 2 = absence of risk factor, 1 = presence of risk factor; bv was coded
0 = no (control) and 1 = yes (case). This coding will give the correct relative risk; the coding used in
Figure 7.12 will not give the same relative risk in SPSS as in Stata.

The output gives two relative risks; the one 'For cohort bv = yes' is the one of interest.

Crosstabs

age * bv Crosstabulation

Row percentages give
the percentage of bv
positive in each group

			bv		Total
			no	yes	
age	<25	Count	116	34	150
		% within age	77.3%	22.7%	100.0%
	>=25	Count	911	140	1051
		% within age	86.7%	13.3%	100.0%
Total		Count	1027	174	1201
		% within age	85.5%	14.5%	100.0%

P value for chi-square
test. If small sample use
Fisher's exact test

Chi-Square Tests

	Value	df	Asymp. Sig. (2-sided)	Exact Sig. (2-sided)	Exact Sig. (1-sided)
Pearson Chi-Square	9.255(b)	1	.002		
Continuity Correction(a)	8.516	1	.004		
Likelihood Ratio	8.295	1	.004		
Fisher's Exact Test				.004	.003
N of Valid Cases	1201				

a Computed only for a 2 x 2 table
b 0 cells (.0%) have expected count less than 5. The minimum expected count is 21.73.

Use two-sided
P value for Fisher's
exact test if small sample

Risk Estimate

	Value	95% Confidence Interval	
		Lower	Upper
Odds Ratio for age (<25 / >=25)	.524	.344	.799
For cohort bv = no	.892	.816	.976
For cohort bv = yes	1.702	1.219	2.375
N of Valid Cases	1201		

If any cells have expected
counts less than 5 then use
Fisher's test

This row: relative risk and
its 95% confidence interval
for having bv (bv = yes)
when under 25 compared
with over 25

Cautionary note The odds ratio and relative risks given here
are reversed in sense and so do not approximate to each other
(see section 7.5.4 for further explanation)

Figure 7.13 Output for chi-squared test and relative risk in SPSS

7.5.4 **Relative risk**

In the early pregnancy study, the risk of bacterial vaginosis could be calculated for all women, and in women with and without various risk factors (Oakeshott *et al.* 2002). Box 5.5 shows the risk of bacterial vaginosis in women under 25 and over 25, and compares them using relative risk. Figures 7.12 and 7.13 show the results of calculating the relative risk in Stata and SPSS. Box 7.10 shows how to present these results within the text. (The same data are also shown in Boxes 5.5 and 5.6, and Figure 5.2.)

From any two-way table it is possible to obtain eight different values for a risk ratio, and so it is important to obtain the right one by coding the variables appropriately. Figures 7.12 and 7.13 show the coding used to produce the correct results. It is fairly simple to check the relative risk by hand by dividing the two proportions on a calculator. We recommend doing this as a way of checking that the program is producing the correct relative risk estimate.

There appears to be an error in SPSS v12 which means that the odds ratios and relative risks do not match up. The odds ratio reported in Figure 7.13 is the odds of having bacterial vaginosis if women are *over* 25 compared with under 25, and shows that the odds are reduced by about 50%. The relative risk, on the other hand, is the risk of having bacterial vaginosis in women *under* 25 compared with over 25, and shows a 70% increase. These results have a similar meaning but the ratios are effectively the inverse of each other.

Note that Stata and SPSS require different coding of the exposure variables to obtain the correct relative risks; details are given in Figures 7.12 and 7.13.

7.5.5 **Odds ratio**

We will illustrate the calculation and presentation of an odds ratio using data from a study of sleepiness in car drivers and car crashes (Connor *et al.* 2002). A total of 529 car drivers involved in crashes where at least one occupant was admitted to hospital or killed ('injury crash'), were compared with 584 car drivers recruited while driving on public roads and representative of all time spent driving in the study region during the study period.

Several variables were analysed, but here we compare the number of drivers who had had less than 5 hours sleep in the 24 hours prior to the crash.

This study was a case–control design where the sample was chosen to have roughly the same number of drivers who had been involved in a crash as who had not. Hence these data cannot be used to

---

BOX 7.10 EXAMPLE

Presenting the results of relative risk

Early Pregnancy Study

Aim of the study To see if miscarriage is associated with bacterial vaginosis.

Study design Cohort study.

Patient population Women booking for antenatal care with general practitioner.

Aim of the analysis To investigate risk factors for bacterial vaginosis.

Description

Methods section

The risk of bacterial vaginosis in women with and without each risk factor is presented and the relative risk used to assess the association of the infection with each risk factor, along with the 95% confidence interval.

Results section

The prevalence of bacterial vaginosis was 23% in women under 25 and 13% in women over 25; relative risk 1.7 (1.2 to 2.4), $P = 0.002$.

Note Box 5.5 shows how the results of several risk factors can be presented in one table.

tab is useful as it keeps the value labels instead of using 'exposed' and 'unexposed' and 'cases' and 'controls'
For **cc** to give correct odds ratio, variables must be coded as 0/1 where 0 = absence of risk factor, 1 = presence
of risk factor; 0 = control and 1 = case
The exposure among cases and controls (row percentages) can be reported but not the risk of disease
(column percentages) as this is a case–control study. **cc** also reports the chi-squared test.

```
. tab case sleep,row chi2

           |         sleep
      case | >5 hours    <=5 hours |     Total
-----------+----------------------+----------
   control |      554          30 |       584
           |    94.86        5.14 |    100.00
-----------+----------------------+----------
      case |      464          65 |       529
           |    87.71       12.29 |    100.00
-----------+----------------------+----------
     Total |     1018          95 |      1113
           |    91.46        8.54 |    100.00

          Pearson chi2(1) =   18.1780    Pr = 0.000
```

P value for chi-squared test

```
. cc case sleep
                                                  Proportion
                  |  Exposed    Unexposed |     Total     Exposed
------------------+----------------------+------------------------
            Cases |       65          464 |       529      0.1229
         Controls |       30          554 |       584      0.0514
------------------+----------------------+------------------------
            Total |       95         1018 |      1113      0.0854
                  |
                  | Point estimate       | [95% Conf. Interval]
                  |----------------------+------------------------
       Odds ratio |      2.586925        |  1.620446    4.202714  (exact)
    Attr. frac. ex. |      .6134407      |   .382886     .7620585  (exact)
    Attr. frac. pop |      .0753755      |
                  +------------------------------------------------
                      chi2(1) =    18.18  Pr>chi2 = 0.0000
```

This row: odds
ratio and 95%
confidence interval

Figure 7.14 Output for odds ratio in Stata

estimate the risk of a crash. While Stata uses commands that will give either a relative risk or an odds ratio, SPSS will always give both but only the odds ratio should be used for a case–control study.

Figures 7.14 and 7.15 show the output from Stata and SPSS for these data, and Box 7.11 shows how this could be presented. The odds of being involved in a crash after less than 5 hours sleep are more than twice the odds when the driver has had 5 hours sleep or more: OR 2.59, 95% CI (1.62 to 4.20), $P < 0.0001$. Note that the confidence limits produced by Stata and SPSS are slightly different because different approximations are used.

7.5.6 Extensions to the two proportion chi-squared test

The chi-squared test for trend is used to look for a trend in ordered proportions. In presenting such data, the same principles apply as used for presenting a comparison of two proportions. It may be appropriate to give the proportions in each category or to use one category as the reference and to show the relative risk or odds ratio for each of the others. Box 7.12 gives an example of presenting such data. The data are from the birthweight study and look for a trend in prevalence of nausea in early pregnancy with smoking.

In Box 7.12 we have given the actual chi-squared test statistic and the degrees of freedom (DF). We recommend doing this for a trend test to distinguish the result from an ordinary chi-squared test on the 2×3 table.

As we discussed before with a simple two-proportion situation (Box 7.9), the choice of presentation depends on the context and personal preference. Confidence intervals could also be added. The nausea data are further analysed, with

Select 'Analyze'
Select 'Descriptive statistics'
Select 'Crosstabs'
Select row and column variables
Select 'Statistics' and tick boxes for 'Chisq' and 'risk' and row percentage
To obtain the correct odds ratio we recommend that variables are coded as 0/1 where 0 = absence of risk factor, 1=presence of risk factor; 0=control and 1=case.
The exposure among cases and controls (row percentages) can be reported but not the risk of disease (column percentages) as this is a case–control study.

case * sleep Crosstabulation

			sleep		Total
			>=5 hours	< 5 hours	
case	no	Count	554	30	584
		% within case	94.9%	5.1%	100.0%
	yes	Count	464	65	529
		% within case	87.7%	12.3%	100.0%
Total		Count	1018	95	1113
		% within case	91.5%	8.5%	100.0%

Chi-squared tests – this table has been omitted here but has the same format as in Figure 7.13

Risk Estimate

	Value	95% Confidence Interval	
		Lower	Upper
Odds Ratio for sleep (0/1)	2.587	1.650	4.056
For cohort case = 0	1.723	1.275	2.329
For cohort case = 1	.666	.572	.776
N of Valid Cases	1113		

Odds ratio and 95% CI SPSS uses a large - sample approximation while Stata uses an exact test

Do not use these

Figure 7.15 Output for odds ratio in SPSS

another factor, using logistic regression later in the book (Box 10.14).

The chi-squared test can also be used on two-way tables with more than two rows and columns. The presentation of the data can then be in proportions (or percentages) calculated either across rows (i.e. so that the row proportion total is 1.0) or down columns (so that the column proportion total is 1.0). The choice of using row or column proportions depends on the context. The overall chi-squared test result can then be given. Further analysis may be done on parts of the table if, and only if, the overall chi-squared test is significant.

Note that all chi-squared tests are large sample tests with the rule of thumb that at least 80% of expected values must be greater than 5 and none are less than 1 for the test to be valid. If the sample is too small, the table can be collapsed by combining rows

---

BOX 7.11 EXAMPLE

Presenting the result of an odds ratio

Road crash study

Aim of the study To investigate risk factors for road crashes.

Study design Case–control study.

Cases Drivers who had been involved in roads crashes.

Controls Drivers who had not been involved in road crashes, recruited whilst driving on public roads.

Description

Methods section

Odds ratios and 95% confidence intervals were calculated to assess the relationship between each risk factor and the risk of being involved in a road traffic crash.

Results section

Of the 529 drivers who had been involved in a road traffic crash, 65 (12%) had had less than 5 hours sleep in the previous 24 hours, compared with 30 out of 584 who had not been involved in a crash. Drivers who have had less than 5 hours sleep were more than twice as likely to be involved in a road traffic crash as those who have had more than 5 hours sleep. Odds ratio 2.6 (1.6 to 4.2), $P < 0.0001$.

Note The interpretation of the odds ratio given above assumes that road traffic crashes are relatively rare and that the odds ratio approximates to the relative risk.

---

and/or columns in an appropriate way. Alternatively, Fisher's exact test can be used, although this may be slow to compute with very large tables and is not available in SPSS for tables larger than 2×2.

7.6 Further reading

All the methods used here are described in standard textbooks of medical statistics and we have not listed all of these. However, we believe that the references given in Box 7.13 are particularly useful for the specific topics discussed in this chapter.

BOX 7.12 EXAMPLE

Example of presenting ordered proportions

Nausea in early pregnancy and smoking in 1511 women

Smoking category	% (nos.) nausea
Non-smoker	83% (845/1021)
Light smoker	73% (246/336)
Heavy smoker	70% (108/154)

Test for trend, $\chi^2 = 21.65$, $P < 0.0001$, DF $= 1$

BOX 7.13 INFORMATION

Useful references to statistical details presented in this chapter

General introduction to confidence intervals and P values
Altman *et al.* (2000, chapter 3), Kirkwood and Sterne (2003, Chapter 8)

Assumptions of the t test
Bland (2000, Chapter 10)

Satterthwaite's modified t test for unequal variances
Armitage *et al.* (2002, Chapter 4) Campbell and Machin (1999, Chapter 7)

Analysing cost data
Thompson and Barber (2000)

Choosing between odds ratios and relative risks
Kirkwood and Sterne (2003, Chapter 16)

Chapter summary

Comparing two groups

- Be selective when reporting results from computer packages as they produce more than is necessary to present or is relevant
- When comparing groups, report summary statistics for each group separately
- Check assumptions of tests used
- Use a transformation, if appropriate, when comparing means
- Give a confidence interval for an estimate of the difference between the two groups (difference in means, difference in proportions, relative risk, or odds ratio)
- Report odds ratios not relative risks for a case–control study even if both are shown on the computer output

CHAPTER 8

Analysing matched or paired data

8.1 Introduction

Matched or paired data can arise in two different ways. The first type of matching arises where two individuals are matched to each other, as in a matched case–control study. In this situation, the two individuals in the matched pair are selected to be as similar to each other as possible apart from the variables being assessed. The variable being assessed is then compared between the pair. For example, in a case–control study investigating school absence after minor injury, 422 children (the cases) who had attended a local emergency department were each matched to a control of the same age, sex, and school. School attendance was compared within the matched pairs (Barnes *et al.* 2001). The second type of matched data arises where two observations or measurements are made on each individual for a particular variable, for example lung function measured before and after exercise to investigate the effects of outdoor air pollution (Hoek *et al.* 1993). Such studies are sometimes known as 'within individual studies'.

It is important to use a statistical method which takes account of the matching when analysing paired data. Paired data are analysed in the same way whether they arise from a matched-pair design or from a within individual design. In this chapter we will consider the unifactorial analysis of both continuous and binary paired data.

Note that the number of controls per case and the number of measurements within individuals need not be limited to two. However, in this chapter we will restrict our attention to the simplest case where there is only one control per case or only two measurements per individual (Box 8.1).

8.2 **Continuous paired data: the paired *t* test**

The data analysed are from the birthweight study. This analysis investigated changes in smoking habit (in smokers only) and caffeine intake during pregnancy (in all women) using serum cotinine and

serum caffeine levels. These blood levels were measured in early and late pregnancy (Cook *et al.* 1996; Peacock *et al.* 1998). Paired *t* tests are used to investigate the changes. Box 8.2 summarises the main features of the test.

The first step in the analysis was to check the distribution of the change in cotinine to ensure that it followed an approximately Normal distribution, as required by the paired *t* test. This showed that the change in cotinine did follow an approximately Normal distribution (Fig. 8.1) The results of this

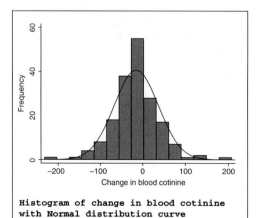

Histogram of change in blood cotinine
with Normal distribution curve

Figure 8.1 Histogram to investigate the distribution of differences in paired data

cotearly and *cotlate* are the cotinine levels in early and late pregnancy. This output gives the mean difference, a *P* value, and a 95% confidence interval for the difference. All means and error terms are given to many more decimal places than required.

Select 'Analyze'

Select 'Compare Means'

Select 'Paired Samples T test'

Move *cotearly* and *cotlate* into 'Paired variables' box

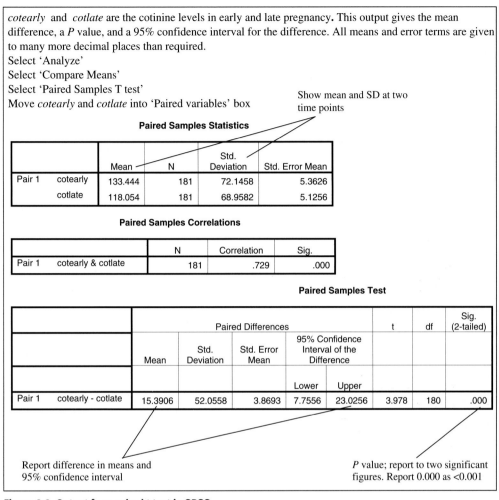

Show mean and SD at two time points

Paired Samples Statistics

		Mean	N	Std. Deviation	Std. Error Mean
Pair 1	cotearly	133.444	181	72.1458	5.3626
	cotlate	118.054	181	68.9582	5.1256

Paired Samples Correlations

		N	Correlation	Sig.
Pair 1	cotearly & cotlate	181	.729	.000

Paired Samples Test

		Paired Differences					t	df	Sig. (2-tailed)
					95% Confidence Interval of the Difference				
		Mean	Std. Deviation	Std. Error Mean	Lower	Upper			
Pair 1	cotearly - cotlate	15.3906	52.0558	3.8693	7.7556	23.0256	3.978	180	.000

Report difference in means and 95% confidence interval

P value; report to two significant figures. Report 0.000 as <0.001

Figure 8.2 Output for a paired t test in SPSS

descriptive analysis would not usually be reported in the main body of a report, particularly if space is limited as is the case in a journal article. However, it might be shown in an appendix if the actual distribution of the variable was of interest.

Giving the individual means and standard deviations allows the reader to see the size and direction of the difference, as well as the variability at the two time points. The results of the paired *t* test using Stata and SPSS are shown in Figures 8.2 and 8.3. Box 8.3 shows how to present the results.

8.2.1 Presenting the results of a paired *t* test

The paired *t* test tests the hypothesis that the difference in means is zero, and so it is appropriate to present the mean and standard deviation at each time point along with the difference and a 95% confidence interval for the difference.

The **ttest** in Stata calculates the changes in cotinine and tests these. It gives the mean difference, a *P* value, and a 95% confidence interval for the difference. All means and error terms are given to many more decimal places than is required.

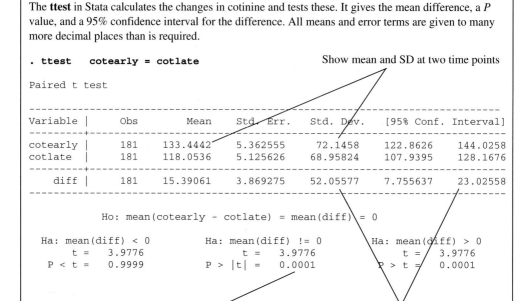

. ttest   cotearly = cotlate   Show mean and SD at two time points

Paired t test

```
--------------------------------------------------------------------------
Variable |    Obs        Mean    Std. Err.   Std. Dev.   [95% Conf. Interval]
---------+----------------------------------------------------------------
cotearly |    181    133.4442    5.362555    72.1458     122.8626    144.0258
 cotlate |    181    118.0536    5.125626    68.95824    107.9395    128.1676
---------+----------------------------------------------------------------
    diff |    181    15.39061    3.869275    52.05577    7.755637    23.02558
--------------------------------------------------------------------------
```

Ho: mean(cotearly - cotlate) = mean(diff) = 0

Ha: mean(diff) < 0   Ha: mean(diff) != 0   Ha: mean(diff) > 0
    t =   3.9776   t =   3.9776   t =   3.9776
P < t =   0.9999   P > |t| =   0.0001   P > t =   0.0001

This *P* value is the two-sided (two-tailed) test   The difference in means and 95%
and is the correct one to use.   confidence interval should be reported

Figure 8.3 Output for a paired t test in Stata

BOX 8.3 EXAMPLE

Presenting the results of a paired *t* test

Birthweight study

Aim of study To investigate smoking, alcohol, and caffeine intake during pregnancy.

Study design Cohort study.

Patient population Consecutive pregnant women booking to deliver their baby at one hospital.

Aim of analysis To compare smoking intake in early and late pregnancy using serum cotinine.

Table. Change in serum cotinine in 181 pregnant smokers between early (approximately 17 weeks gestation) and late (36 weeks) pregnancy

	Mean (SD)		Difference (95% CI)	P value
	Early	Late	(early-late)	
Cotinine (ng/ml)	133.4 (72.1)	118.0 (69.0)	15.4 (7.8 to 23.0)	0.0001

Description

Methods section

Changes in serum cotinine were examined using a paired *t* test.

Results section

Mean cotinine level decreased by a small but statistically significant amount (15.4 ng/ml) between early and late pregnancy (table).

(Peacock *et al.* 1998)

8.2.2 **Log transformations**

Figure 8.4 shows the distribution of the change in serum caffeine over pregnancy. The figure shows that these data are positively skewed, but that they are approximately Normal after logarithmic transformation. Therefore the transformed data were

analysed using the paired *t* test. As for the two-sample *t* test, transforming the data changes the hypothesis being tested (Box 8.4). Note that the raw data are transformed, i.e. the data are transformed, *before* differences are calculated.

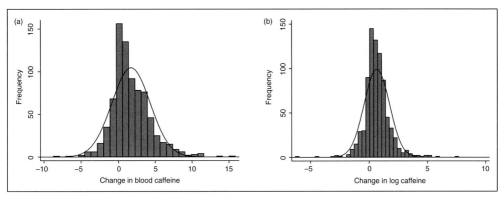

Figure 8.4 Histogram of skewed paired data (a) before and (b) after log transformation with Normal distribution curve

---

BOX 8.5 EXAMPLE

Presenting the results of a paired *t* test on log-transformed data

Birthweight study

Aim of study To investigate smoking, alcohol, and caffeine intake during pregnancy.

Study design Cohort study.

Patient population: Consecutive pregnant women booking to deliver their baby at one hospital.

Aim of analysis To compare changes in caffeine intake during pregnancy in 801 pregnant women using serum caffeine.

Table. Change in serum caffeine in pregnant women between early (approximately 17 weeks gestation) and late (36 weeks) pregnancy.

	Geometric mean (95% CI)		Ratio of geometric means (early/late)	
	Early	**Late**	**(95% CI)**	**P value**
Caffeine (ng/ml)	1.60 (1.48, 1.73)	3.02 (2.84, 3.22)	0.53 (0.49, 0.57)	<0.0001

Description

Methods section

The differences in serum caffeine were positively skew and so the raw data were log-transformed. This gave differences which followed an approximately Normal distribution. The paired *t* test was used with the transformed data and results presented as the ratio of geometric means and 95% confidence intervals.

Results section

Mean serum caffeine level in early pregnancy was approximately half of that in late pregnancy and this change was highly significant (table).

(Cook *et al.* 1996)

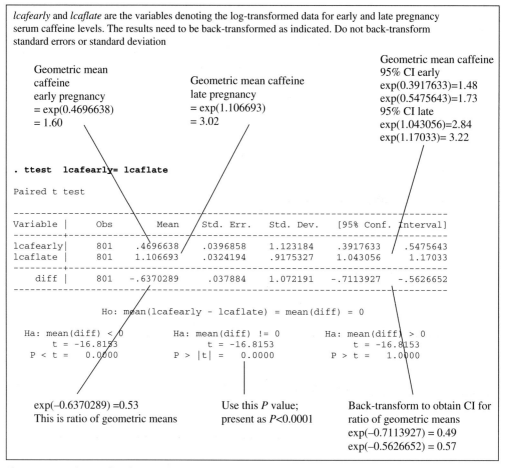

lcafearly and *lcaflate* are the variables denoting the log-transformed data for early and late pregnancy serum caffeine levels. The results need to be back-transformed as indicated. Do not back-transform standard errors or standard deviation

Geometric mean caffeine early pregnancy = exp(0.4696638) = 1.60

Geometric mean caffeine late pregnancy = exp(1.106693) = 3.02

Geometric mean caffeine 95% CI early
exp(0.3917633)=1.48
exp(0.5475643)=1.73
95% CI late
exp(1.043056)=2.84
exp(1.17033)= 3.22

```
. ttest  lcafearly= lcaflate

Paired t test

------------------------------------------------------------------------------
Variable |    Obs       Mean    Std. Err.   Std. Dev.   [95% Conf. Interval]
---------+--------------------------------------------------------------------
lcafearly|    801    .4696638   .0396858   1.123184    .3917633    .5475643
lcaflate |    801   1.106693    .0324194   .9175327    1.043056    1.17033
---------+--------------------------------------------------------------------
    diff |    801   -.6370289   .037884    1.072191    -.7113927   -.5626652
------------------------------------------------------------------------------
           Ho: mean(lcafearly - lcaflate) = mean(diff) = 0

 Ha: mean(diff) < 0         Ha: mean(diff) != 0         Ha: mean(diff) > 0
    t = -16.8153              t = -16.8153                 t = -16.8153
 P < t =   0.0000         P > |t| =   0.0000           P > t =   1.0000
```

exp(−0.6370289) =0.53
This is ratio of geometric means

Use this *P* value; present as *P*<0.0001

Back-transform to obtain CI for ratio of geometric means
exp(−0.7113927) = 0.49
exp(−0.5626652) = 0.57

Figure 8.5 Back-transforming a paired t test output from Stata

---

BOX 8.4 INFORMATION

The paired *t* test on log-transformed data

Null hypothesis The ratio of the population geometric means at the two time points equals 1.

Use for continuous variables with a positive skew.

Assumptions The differences after transformation follow a Normal distribution.

Note The standard deviations and standard errors cannot be back-transformed, but confidence intervals can.

8.2.3 Presenting the results after log transformation

The Stata and SPSS outputs are shown in Figures 8.5 and 8.6. The key points to note are that the standard deviations and standard errors on the log scale cannot

be back-transformed to the natural scale and so other measures of spread or precision have to be used. Therefore we recommend presenting the individual back-transformed means and their 95% confidence intervals which give meaningful values on the original natural scale. As we have shown previously in chapters 5 and 7, the back-transformed means are no longer arithmetic means but are the geometric means, and the back-transformed difference is the ratio of geometric means (Box 8.5).

8.2.4 Comment on results

The high peakedness of the caffeine distribution (Fig. 8.4) was due to the women whose intake changed little over pregnancy (there were four women whose intake did not change at all). It is likely that the lower caffeine intake in early pregnancy was a result of nausea and vomiting which is very common during the first trimester of pregnancy.

lcafearly and *lcaflate* are the caffeine levels in early and late pregnancy. This output gives the mean difference, a *P* value, and a 95% confidence interval for the difference. The results need to be back-transformed as indicated. Do not back-transform standard errors or standard deviations.

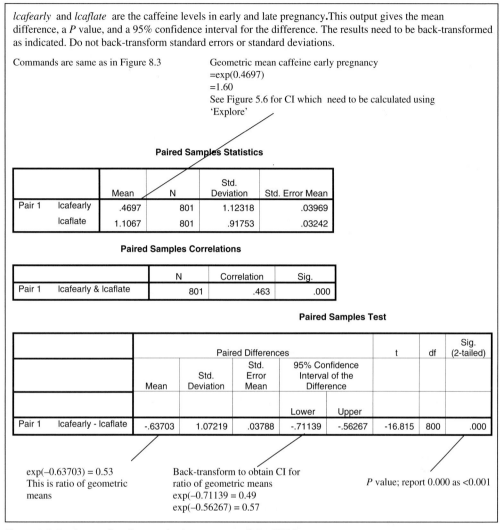

Commands are same as in Figure 8.3

Geometric mean caffeine early pregnancy
=exp(0.4697)
=1.60
See Figure 5.6 for CI which need to be calculated using 'Explore'

Paired Samples Statistics

		Mean	N	Std. Deviation	Std. Error Mean
Pair 1	lcafearly	.4697	801	1.12318	.03969
	lcaflate	1.1067	801	.91753	.03242

Paired Samples Correlations

		N	Correlation	Sig.
Pair 1	lcafearly & lcaflate	801	.463	.000

Paired Samples Test

		Paired Differences					t	df	Sig. (2-tailed)
		Mean	Std. Deviation	Std. Error Mean	95% Confidence Interval of the Difference				
					Lower	Upper			
Pair 1	lcafearly - lcaflate	-.63703	1.07219	.03788	-.71139	-.56267	-16.815	800	.000

exp(−0.63703) = 0.53
This is ratio of geometric means

Back-transform to obtain CI for ratio of geometric means
exp(−0.71139 = 0.49
exp(−0.56267) = 0.57

P value; report 0.000 as <0.001

Figure 8.6 Back-transforming a paired *t* test output from SPSS

8.2.5 Extending the analysis

These data could be used to explore further the changes in smoking and caffeine across pregnancy by investigating whether changes in smoking and caffeine are explained by symptoms; for example, women often drink less coffee in early pregnancy because they suffer from morning sickness. To investigate this we would use multiple regression which allows us to model the effect of one variable on an outcome, after allowing for the effect of another (see Chapter 10).

8.3 Non-Normal data

The example is taken from a small study of sleep in newborn babies who were laid to sleep in two different positions, each for a specified length of time. Various observations were recorded in the two sleep positions, including the number of awakenings (defined according to a protocol). The difference in number of awakenings between the two positions did not follow a Normal distribution and a logarithmic transformation did not improve matters, and so the sign test was used.

The first step was to compute summary statistics (the median and range for the number of awakenings while sleeping in two different positions) and then to use the sign test. Box 8.6 gives some further information about the test.

8.3.1 Presenting the results of non-parametric or rank tests

The Stata and SPSS outputs are shown in Figures 8.7 and 8.8. The limitation of these tests as opposed to the *t* test is that they are essentially significance tests and do not provide easily interpretable estimates. Therefore some summary statistics need to be calculated and presented alongside the *P* value to allow the result of the test to be interpreted. We have presented the median, interquartile range, and full range here (Box 8.7). In other situations, either the interquartile range or the range may be sufficient.

BOX 8.6 INFORMATION

Sign test for matched pairs

Null hypothesis The probability of a positive difference equals the probability of a negative difference.

Most suitable for
◆ Ordered categorical data, scores.
◆ Discrete or continuous data that cannot be transformed to a symmetrical distribution.

Assumptions Differences within individuals can be rated as positive or negative.

Not suitable for situations where many differences are zero.

Limitations
◆ Need at least six observations (pairs) for statistical significance to be possible.
◆ Significance test only.

---

awake1 and *awake2* are the two variables for the number of awakenings in each position

Stata gives the one-sided as well as the two-sided result. The two-sided *P* value should be used. Note that summary statistics would be calculated before doing the test. These are not shown here.

```
. gen diffawakening= awake1-awake2

. signtest   diffawakenings=0

Sign test

           sign |    observed       expected
  --------------+-----------------------------
       positive |        2            11.5
       negative |       21            11.5
           zero |        1             1
  --------------+-----------------------------
            all |       24            24

One-sided tests:
  Ho: median of diffawak~s = 0 vs.
  Ha: median of diffawak~s > 0
        Pr(#positive >= 2) =
            Binomial(n = 23, x >= 2, p = 0.5)  =   1.0000

  Ho: median of diffawak~s = 0 vs.
  Ha: median of diffawak~s < 0
        Pr(#negative >= 21) =
            Binomial(n = 23, x >= 21, p = 0.5)  =   0.0000

Two-sided test:
  Ho: median of diffawak~s = 0 vs.
  Ha: median of diffawak~s != 0
        Pr(#positive >= 21 or #negative >= 21) =
      min(1, 2*Binomial(n = 23, x >= 21, p = 0.5))  =   0.0001
```

Use this two-sided *P* value

Figure 8.7 Output for a sign test from Stata

awake1 and *awake2* are the two variables for the number of awakenings in each position.
Select 'Analyze'
Select 'Non parametric Tests'
Select '2 Related Samples'
Move *awake1*and *awake2* to 'Test Pair(s) List'
Tick box for 'Sign test'

Frequencies

		N
awake1 awake2	Negative Differences(a)	2
	Positive Differences(b)	21
	Ties(c)	1
	Total	24

a awake1 < awake2
b awake1 > awake2
c awake1 = awake2

Test Statistics(b)

	awake1-awake2
Exact Sig. (2-tailed)	.000(a)

a Binomial distribution used.
b Sign Test

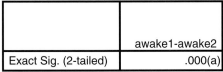 *P* value for sign test;
report as *P*<0.001

Figure 8.8 Output for a sign test from SPSS

BOX 8.7 EXAMPLE

Presenting the findings of a sign test

Sleep study

Aim of study To investigate the differences in various sleep parameters according to sleeping position.
Study design within individual intervention study.
Patient population Twenty-four newborn babies.
Aim of analysis To compare the number of awakenings in two sleep positions, 1 and 2.

Table. Comparison of number of awakenings according to sleep position in 24 babies

Position	Median	Interquartile range	Min, Max	P value
1	36.5	30 to 40	12, 48	
2	18.5	15 to 25	10, 35	
Difference	15.5	−8.5 to 21.5	−22, 36	<0.0001

Description

Methods section
The difference in number of awakenings in the two sleeping positions was calculated for each baby. Since the differences followed an irregular distribution, they were compared using the sign test.

Results section
The median number of awakenings was approximately twice as high for position 1 than for position 2, and this difference was highly significant (table).

Note The median of the differences (15.5) is not the same as the difference in medians (36.5 − 18.5 = 18).

8.4 **Matched case–control data**

The data analysed here are from a case–control study of bronchodilator treatment and death from asthma. The cases were patients who had died from asthma, and the controls were patients admitted to hospital for asthma (Anderson *et al.* 2005). Controls were one-to-one matched for period, age, and area. We will analyse three drugs here (short-acting β agonists, oral steroids, and antibiotics) to illustrate the methodology and the presentation of the data. We will only show the Stata and SPSS outputs for one treatment, short-acting β agonists, since the principle is the same for all three (Figs. 8.9 and 8.10).

McNemar's test (Box 8.8) is used to test the hypothesis that the proportion exposed to the drug is the same in the cases and controls. The strength of association is estimated by the conditional odds ratio.

BOX 8.8 INFORMATION

McNemar's test

Null hypothesis The population prevalence is the same under two conditions.

Use this test for two paired proportions when:

◆ Testing the hypothesis that the underlying prevalence of an exposure is the same in cases and controls.

◆ Testing the hypothesis that the underlying prevalence of a condition is the same at two time points.

◆ Testing the hypothesis that the underlying prevalence of a condition is the same under two experimental situations in a cross-over study.

Do not use this test when:

◆ Testing the hypothesis that one variable is related to another.

◆ Comparing unpaired proportions in a case–control study

Use the ordinary chi-squared test for these situation.

BOX 8.9 HELPFUL TIPS

Calculating conditional odds ratios for SPSS users

SPSS v12 will only calculate McNemar's test and produce the table. The following method uses the 95% confidence interval for a single proportion (section 6.2) to calculate the 95% confidence interval for the conditional odds ratio.

Suppose

◆ s denotes the number of pairs where the case is exposed to the risk factor and the control is not.

◆ t denotes the numbers of pairs where the control is exposed to the risk factor and the case is not.

Then

◆ The conditional odds ratio $= s/t$.

◆ $s/(s+t)$ is the proportion of discordant pairs where case is exposed.

◆ $s/(s+t)$ is a proportion and the 95% confidence interval can be calculated using **biconf** (www-users.york.ac.uk). Alternatively, **CIPROPORTION** (www.cardiff.ac.uk) could be used as in Figure 6.2 but will give slightly different confidence limits to Stata (see section 6.2).

◆ If p_L and p_U denote the lower and upper limits of the confidence interval for $s/(s+t)$, then the confidence interval for the conditional odds ratio is given by

$$p_L/(1-p_L) \text{ to } p_U/(1-p_U).$$

Figure 8.9 gives a worked example.

This is not available in SPSS, but can be calculated using any program that will calculate a confidence interval for a single proportion such a **biconf**, which is available free (Box 2.8), or CIPROPORTION as in Figure 6.2. The details of the method are given in Box 8.9 and a worked example is shown in Figure 8.10.

Note that the calculations shown in Figure 8.10 gives the proportion with the risk factor in the cases and controls, whereas the output in Figure 8.12 uses frequencies.

case and *control* are the variables which denote the presence or absence of β_2-agonist use in the cases and controls. The data are coded 1/0 for β_2-agonist use yes/no, and are labelled as exposed and unexposed.

Select 'Analyze'
Select 'Descriptive Statistics'
Select 'Crosstabs'
Select row and column variables
Select 'Statistics' and tick box for 'McNemar'. Do not select the risk option to calculate the odds ratio.

case * controlCrosstabulation

Count

		control		Total
		Unexposed	Exposed	
case	Unexposed	7	45	52
Total	Exposed	69	411	480
		76	456	532

Chi-SquareTests

	Value	Exact Sig. (2-sided)
McNemar Test		.031(a)
N of Valid Cases	532	

a Binomial distribution used.

Calculating the conditional odds ratio and 95% confidence interval

Using notation in Box 8.9, $s = 69$ and $t = 45$

Conditional odds ratio $= s/t = 69/45 = 1.533$

Number of cases exposed among discordant pairs is 69 and total number of discordant pairs is 114

Using biconf (www-users.york.ac.uk), where number of trials is 114 and number of successes is 69, gives 95% CI as 0.50937to 0.69553

95% confidence interval for odds ratio is 0.50937/(1–0.50937) to 0.69553/(1–0.69553), i.e. 1.038 to 2.284

Figure 8.9 Output for a matched case–control analysis in SPSS

case and *control* are the variables which denote the presence or absence of β_2-agonist use in the cases and controls. This is expressed as 'exposed' and unexposed' in Stata. The data are coded 1/0 for β_2-agonist use yes/no.

Note that Stata gives two *P* values, one derived from the chi-squared distribution and an exact one. We recommend using the exact one since, if the sample is small the chi-squared *P* value may be too small, and if the sample is large there will be little difference between the two values.

```
. mcc case control
```

```
                | Controls                    |
Cases           |  Exposed    Unexposed  |      Total
----------------+------------------------+-----------
      Exposed |     411           69  |        480
    Unexposed |      45            7  |         52
----------------+------------------------+-----------
        Total |     456           76  |        532
```

McNemar's chi2(1) =   5.05   Prob > chi2 = 0.0246   Use this *P*
Exact McNemar significance probability   = 0.0308 ——— value
Proportion with factor
        Cases   .9022556
        Controls   .8571429   [95% Conf. Interval]
                       ---------   --------------------
        difference   .0451128   .0040844   .0861411
        ratio   1.052632   1.006585   1.100785
        rel. diff.   .3157895   .0880272   .5435518

        odds ratio   1.533333   1.038233   2.28449   (exact)

Use this odds ratio and 95% CI

Figure 8.10 Output for a matched case–control analysis in Stata

8.4.1 Presentation of matched case–control data

The results are presented in Box 8.10. We have shown the percentage of cases and controls that were exposed, as well as the conditional odds ratios, 95% confidence intervals, and *P* values. Note that one *P* value is very large, and was given in the Stata output as '1.0000', meaning that it is 1 when rounded to four decimal places. We have presented this as >0.999 (see Box 5.1).

We have described the association in terms of increased or reduced risk, as appropriate, and have quoted the actual odds ratio. This will approximate to the relative risk since the outcome (death from asthma) is rare, but we have referred to this as the

'odds ratio' throughout as a reminder that the odds ratio and relative risk are not exactly the same thing.

8.4.2 Comment on results and extensions

The treatments presented here are only a small subset of all those analysed and the majority of treatments were not significantly associated with death. The published paper discussed the clinical significance of these statistically significant findings. In addition, the authors adjusted their odds ratios for sex using conditional logistic regression. This did not affect the results substantially (see Anderson *et al.* (2005) for more details).

BOX 8.10 EXAMPLE

Presenting the results of a matched case–control analysis

Asthma case–control study

Aim of study To investigate the effects of long- to medium-term drug treatment for asthma.

Study design Matched case–control study.

Patient population 532 patients aged 64 or less who died from asthma and 532 matched controls who were hospitalised for asthma. Matching was for period, age, and area.

Aim of analysis To investigate the relationship between bronchodilator treatment and death from asthma.

Table. Odds ratios (95% confidence intervals) for death associated with treatment 1–5 years before the index date in 532 matched case–control pairs

Drug	case (%)[1]	control (%)	Odds ratio (95%CI)	P value
Short-acting β_2 agonist	90%	86%	1.53 (1.04 to 2.28)	0.031
Oral steroids	72%	72%	1.01 (0.77 to 1.33)	>0.999
Antibiotics	86%	90%	0.66 (0.44 to 0.97)	0.032

[1] Proportion exposed to drug in case and control groups.

Description

Methods section

The exposure to drug treatment in cases and controls was compared using McNemar's test. The results are presented as matched odds ratios and 95% confidence intervals.

Results section

Exposure to short-acting β_2 agonists, oral steroids, and antibiotics was high in cases and controls. The prescription of short-acting β_2 agonists was associated with a significantly increased risk of asthma death with an odds ratio of 1.53. Antibiotic use was associated with a significantly reduced risk of death with an odds ratio of 0.66. There was no evidence for any effect of oral steroids (table). (Anderson *et al.* 2005)

8.5 **Matched cohort data**

The data analysed are again from the birthweight study. This analysis investigated the prevalence of various symptoms reported by the women in early and late pregnancy and sought to quantify the changes in symptoms that occurred as pregnancy progressed. This was of interest because it was thought that some symptoms were common in early pregnancy and then declined in prevalence, whereas other symptoms became more common as pregnancy progressed (Meyer *et al.* 1994).

The first step in the analysis was to look at the frequency of each symptom at the two time points alone. Secondly, the symptoms were cross-tabulated at the two time points to see how many women reported the symptom at both, neither, or one time point only.

McNemar's test is used to test the changes in prevalence and the results are given as ratios of proportions and *P* values. McNemar's test is testing the null hypothesis that the prevalence of symptoms does not change over pregnancy (Box 8.8).

Eleven symptoms were analysed in the study. Results will be given for all, but details of the outputs from Stata and SPSS will only be given for a selection since the principle is the same for all.

Note that the change in prevalence over pregnancy could be presented as the difference of proportions rather than the ratio of proportions. We chose to use the ratio since we were interested in the relative change in prevalence rather than the absolute change. In other situations the difference may be a more appropriate summary of the changes (see Bland 2000, Chapter 13, section 13.9).

Nausea in early and late pregnancy are given by *nausea1* and *nausea2*. The Stata command **mcc** performs matched chi-squared tests. Because the Stata output is presented in the format for a case–control design, using 'exposed' and 'unexposed',we have also produced the simple cross-tabulation to show which cells refer to the symptom combinations 'yes/yes', 'no/no', etc. The data were coded 0/1 for no/yes.

The ratio of proportions is the ratio of the prevalence of the symptom at the two time points. Note that the odds ratio given in the Stata output should be ignored asthisis not a case–control study.

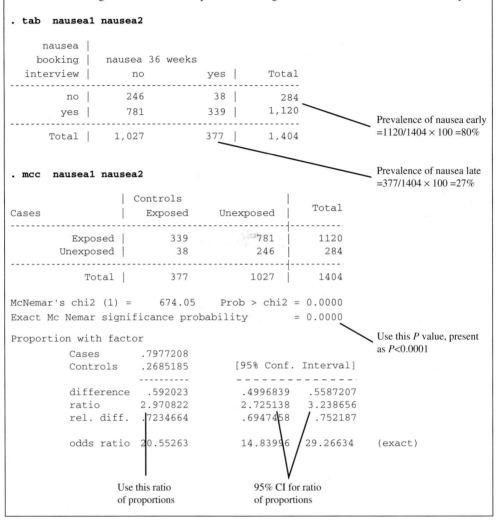

. **tab**   **nausea1 nausea2**

nausea booking interview	nausea 36 weeks no	yes	Total
no	246	38	284
yes	781	339	1,120
Total	1,027	377	1,404

Prevalence of nausea early =1120/1404 × 100 =80%

. **mcc**   **nausea1 nausea2**

Cases	Controls Exposed	Unexposed	Total
Exposed	339	781	1120
Unexposed	38	246	284
Total	377	1027	1404

Prevalence of nausea late =377/1404 × 100 =27%

McNemar's chi2 (1) =   674.05   Prob > chi2 = 0.0000
Exact Mc Nemar significance probability   = 0.0000

Proportion with factor

		[95% Conf. Interval]
Cases	.7977208	
Controls	.2685185	
difference	.592023	.4996839 .5587207
ratio	2.970822	2.725138 3.238656
rel. diff.	.7234664	.6947458 .752187
odds ratio	20.55263	14.83996 29.26634 (exact)

Use this *P* value, present as *P*<0.0001

Use this ratio of proportions

95% CI for ratio of proportions

Figure 8.11 Output for McNemar's test with ratio of paired proportions in Stata

The ratio of proportions is calculated in Stata (Fig. 8.11) but is not available in SPSS v12.

The disadvantage of using the ratio of prevalences is that the methodology for estimating a confidence interval is recent (Nam and Blackwelder 2002) and so is not routinely available. Stata will estimate the confidence interval but SPSS will not at the time of writing this book. Therefore we have chosen to omit the confidence interval from the presentation but have indicated it on the Stata output. Box 8.11 summarises the ways of presenting paired proportions.

Nausea in early and late pregnancy are given by *nausea1* and *nausea2*. The data were coded 0/1 for no/yes.
Select 'Analyze'
Select 'Descriptive Statistics'
Select 'Frequencies'
Select variables *nausea1* and *nausea2*

Select 'Analyze'
Select 'Descriptive statistics'
Select 'Crosstabs'
Select row and column variables
Select 'Statistics' and tick box for 'McNemar'. Do not select the risk option to calculate the relative risk

nausea atbooking interview

		Frequency	Percent	Valid Percent	Cumulative Percent
Valid	no	284	20.2	20.2	20.2
	yes	1120	79.8	79.8	100.0
	Total	1404	100.0	100.0	

Ratio of prevalences of nausea
= 79.8/26.9
= 2.97

nauseas 36 weeks

		Frequency	Percent	Valid Percent	Cumulative Percent
Valid	no	1027	73.1	73.1	73.1
	yes	377	26.9	26.9	100.0
	Total	1404	100.0	100.0	

nausea at booking interview * nauseas 36 weeks Crosstabulation

Count

		nauseas 36 weeks		Total
		no	yes	
nausea at booking interview	no	246	38	284
	yes	781	339	1120
Total		1027	377	1404

Chi-Square Tests

	Value	Exact Sig. (2-sided)
McNemar Test		.000(a)
N of Valid Cases	1404	
a Binomial distribution used.		

P value for McNemar's test, present as *P*<0.001

Figure 8.12 Output for cross-tabulation and McNemar's test with ratio of paired proportions in SPSS

BOX 8.11 SUMMARY

Presenting paired proportions

Matched case–control study
Conditional (matched) odds ratio and 95% CI.

Matched cohort data
Difference of proportions and 95% CI.
or
Ratio of proportions and 95% CI.*
*Note This is a new method and the CI is not routinely available but can be done in Stata

8.5.1 Presenting the results of a matched cohort study

The Stata and SPSS outputs are shown in Figures 8.11 and 8.12. We recommend doing an ordinary tabulation before performing the test to make sure that it is clear which way round the package has presented the results. Stata can be confusing because it uses the terminology of a case–control study whenever McNemar's test is used.

There was no obvious ordering to the symptoms and so we have presented them in descending order

BOX 8.12 EXAMPLE

Presenting the findings for a matched cohort study

Birthweight Study

Aim of analysis To investigate symptoms and health problems in pregnancy.

Study design Cohort study.

Patient population 1404 pregnant women booking in one hospital.

Aim of analysis To compare the prevalence of common symptoms across pregnancy.

Table. Prevalence of symptoms in early(approx, 17 weeks) and late (36 weeks) pregnancy in 1404 women

Symptom	Prevalence in pregnancy		Ratio of prevalances	P value
	Early %	**Late** %		
Nausea	80	27	3.0	<0.0001
Breast tenderness	80	26	3.1	<0.0001
Vomiting	46	17	2.7	<0.0001
Backache	45	68	0.66	<0.0001
Felt faint	40	21	1.9	<0.0001
Constipation	40	20	2.0	<0.0001
Indigestion	36	72	0.50	<0.0001
Diarrhoea	13	16	0.79	0.0049
Haemorrhoids	11	17	0.66	<0.0001
Varicose veins	9.3	13	0.73	0.0001
Actually fainted	5.9	1.2	4.9	<0.0001

Note that the symptoms have been ordered by prevalence at the first time point.

Description

Methods section
The prevalence of symptoms at two points in pregnancy was compared using McNemar's test. Results were presented as ratios of prevalence.

Results section
The distribution of symptoms was markedly different for early and late pregnancy. The most common symptoms in early pregnancy were nausea and breast tenderness, which were reported by most women. The most common symptoms in late pregnancy were indigestion and backache, which were reported by more than two-thirds of women. Many symptoms, including nausea and breast tenderness, declined dramatically in prevalence over pregnancy. Conversely, indigestion, backache, and haemorrhoids all became more common as pregnancy progressed. All changes, whether increase or decrease in prevalence, were highly statistically significant.

(Meyer *et al.* 1994)

of prevalence (Box 8.12). Since the study was a longitudinal design rather than case–control, the ratio of prevalences can be calculated directly and these have been presented rather than using odds (see section 8.4).

8.5.2 Comment on results

The results show the varying patterns of different symptoms across pregnancy. It may be that the changes in smoking and caffeine across pregnancy are related to these symptoms.

Nausea in pregnancy is common, with more than 50% of women experiencing the symptom early in pregnancy, and so the odds ratio will not approximate to the relative risk. Figure 8.11 gives the odds ratio as 20.6 while the relative risk is only 3.0. If the odds ratio is interpreted as if it were the relative risk, then it would give a gross overestimate of the strength of the relationship. For further discussion see Davies *et al.* (1998).

8.6 **Further reading**

The references given in Box 8.13 are those that we have found particularly useful for the specific topics listed.

BOX 8.13 INFORMATION

Further information on statistical methods

Paired t tests

Altman (1991, Chapter 9), Armitage *et al.* (2002, Chapter 4), Bland (2000, Chapter 10), Campbell and Machin (1999, Chapter 6), Kirkwood and Sterne (2003, Chapter 7)

Wilcoxon signed rank test, sign test

Altman (1991, Chapter 9), Armitage *et al.* (2002, Chapter 10), Bland (2000, Chapters 9, 12), Kirkwood and Sterne (2003, Chapter 30)

McNemar's test

Altman (1991, Chapter 10), Armitage *et al.* (2002, Chapter 4), Bland (2000, Chapter 13), Kirkwood and Sterne (2003, Chapter 21)

Transformations

Altman (1991, Chapter 7), Armitage *et al.* (2002, Chapter 10), Bland (2000, Chapter 10), Kirkwood and Sterne (2003, Chapter 13)

Matched case-control data

Altman (1991, Chapter 10), Campbell and Machin (1999, Chapter 9), Kirkwood and Sterne (2003, Chapter 21)

Paired odds ratio

Altman *et al.* (2000, Chapter 7), Bland (2000, Chapter 13)

Risk difference for paired proportions

Altman et al. (2000, Chapter 7), Bland (2000, Chapter 13)

Chapter summary

Analysing paired data

◆ Analyse paired data using a method which takes the pairing into account

◆ Present summary statistics (e.g. means, proportions) for the two groups or two time periods, as appropriate, giving some indication of scatter or spread for ordinal data

◆ Present a summary statistic (e.g. difference in means, difference in proportions, odds ratio, relative risk) and 95% confidence interval for the association or change within the pairs wherever possible

◆ Describe the size and direction of the findings as well as the statistical significance

CHAPTER 9

Analysing relationships between variables

9.1 Introduction

Correlation analysis can be used to investigate the strength of the relationship between two continuous variables. For example, in the birthweight study we wanted to see how the baby's birthweight, head circumference, crown–heel length, and upper arm circumference were related to each other. Correlation analysis gives a single index, the correlation coefficient, which summarises how strong the relationship is (Box 9.1).

Another situation arises if we want to investigate the nature of the relationship between two variables. For example, how much does peak flow rate in children increase with age? This question can be answered by regression analysis.

With regression analysis, we regard one variable as the 'outcome' and the other as a potential 'predictor' or 'explanatory' variable. In the example of peak flow rate and age, the outcome is peak flow rate and the explanatory variable is age because we are investigating how peak flow rate changes with age. Specifically, do older children have higher peak flows, and if they do, how much does peak flow increase with age? Analyses of this kind are performed using simple linear regression (Box 9.1).

9.2 Correlation

Pearson's correlation coefficient is the standard method for assessing the strength of the relationship between two variables and is closely aligned to linear regression. The assumptions are described in Box 9.2. Other methods, Spearman's rho and

When to use correlation and regression

Correlation

◆ Investigates strength of relationship between two ordinal variables

◆ Neither variable can be assumed to predict the other

◆ For example, baby's birthweight and head circumference—how closely are they related?

◆ Gives a single index—the correlation coefficient

Regression

◆ Investigates nature of relationship between two continuous variables

◆ One variable is the outcome; the other is the predictor or explanatory variable

◆ Want to know how much the outcome changes when the predictor changes

◆ For example, peak flow rate (outcome) and child's age (predictor)—by how much does mean peak flow rate increase as child's age increases?

◆ Gives the equation of the line (slope and intercept) which can be used for prediction, i.e. to predict the mean peak flow rate for a given age

Pearson's correlation

Also known as the product–moment correlation coefficient.

Null hypothesis There is no linear (straight-line) relationship between the two variables in the population.

Assumptions for a significance test At least one of the two variables follows a Normal distribution.

Deviations from assumptions

◆ Try transforming one or both variables, as appropriate

◆ If transformation is not possible, use a rank method: either Spearman's rank or Kendall's tau coefficient

Checking assumptions

◆ Plot data to show the shape and direction of relationship

◆ May be able to see if data are approximately Normal from scatterplot. Alternatively, use histograms or Normal plots

Confidence intervals

◆ Both variables must be Normally distributed to calculate the confidence interval

---

Kendall's tau-b (section 9.2.6), are based on the ranks of the data rather than on the data values themselves, and can be used if the assumptions for Pearson's method do not hold.

9.2.1 Pearson's correlation coefficient

In this example we will use data from the UKOS validation study (Box 6.2). We wanted to know how strong the relationship was between two scores, both measuring the mental development of the child. The mental development index, obtained from clinical assessment, was the gold standard and was compared with the parental questionnaire score. These were measured on different scales. To investigate how strongly the two measures were related, first the data were plotted and then the product–moment correlation was calculated.

The graph in Box 9.3 shows the scatterplot. From this we can see a reasonably strong positive relationship. There is no obvious curvature and it would seem reasonable to fit a straight line to the data in the graph.

9.2.2 Presenting the results of a correlation analysis

Sometimes the value for a single correlation coefficient is given with a scatterplot and sometimes it is simply stated in the text (Box 9.3). Summary statistics for the two variables should be given as well as the actual correlation as shown in Box 9.3.

Figures 9.1 and 9.2 show the Stata and SPSS outputs. To calculate the confidence interval in Stata using the raw data, the command **ci2** needs to be downloaded from the Stata website (www.stata.com).

BOX 9.3 EXAMPLE

Presenting the results for Pearson's correlation

UKOS validation study

Aim of study To validate a new screening tool for cognitive function in children.

Study design Cross-sectional screening study.

Patient population Sixty-four parents and their children aged 2 years who were born very prematurely.

Aim of analysis To calculate the correlation between the mental development index and the parental questionnaire score.

Description

Methods section

The strength of relationship between the mental development index (MDI) and the parental questionnaire score was estimated by the product–moment correlation coefficient.

Results section

Table. Summary statistics for MDI and parental questionnaire score

	No.	Mean	SD	Min	Max
MDI	64	81	19	50	120
Parental questionnaire score	64	70	35	3	142

Sixty-four children were included in the study. There was a wide spread of scores and the mean MDI was below the expected mean of 100 (table). There was a moderately strong, positive correlation between the MDI and parental score ($r=0.68$, $P<0.001$).

Alternative presentation of correlation in scatterplot (the same description could be used)

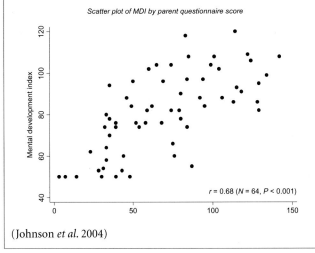

(Johnson *et al.* 2004)

To calculate it from summary data, the immediate command **cii2** can be used (see Fig. 9.1).

SPSS does not give a confidence interval for the correlation coefficient and so if one is required then the user has to use another package such as Clinstat (www-users.york.ac.uk) or CIA (www.som.soton.ac.uk) or use the formulae given in a textbook (Bland 2000; Petrie and Sabin 2000; Altman 1991; Altman *et al.* 2000; Kirkwood and Sterne 2003). Helpful tips for reporting correlations are given in Box 9.4.

mdi is the mental development index score and *parent* is the parental questionnaire score. Note that we calculate the summary statistics before calculating the correlation.

```
. sum  mdi parent

    Variable |        Obs        Mean    Std. Dev.        Min        Max
-------------+--------------------------------------------------------
         mdi |         64      81.375    18.94897          50        120
      parent |         64    69.53125    34.99704           3        142

. pwcorr  mdi parent, sig

             |      mdi    parent
-------------+------------------
         mdi |   1.0000
             |
      parent |   0.6798    1.0000
             |   0.0000
             |
. ci2   mdi parent,corr

Confidence interval for Pearson's product-moment correlation
of mdi and parent based on Fisher's transformation.
Correlation = 0.680 on 64 observations (95% CI: 0.521 to 0.793)
```

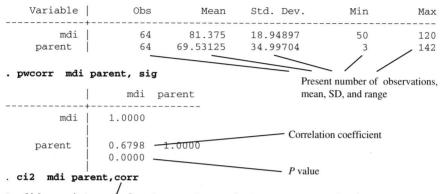

Present number of observations, mean, SD, and range

Correlation coefficient

P value

To calculate CIs from raw data **ci2** needs to be downloaded from the Stata website (www.stata.com). From the help menu search for **ci2** and install.

Note that the immediate command is available in Stata but the user has to enter the summary data, sample size, and correlation: **cii2 64 0.6798, corr**. This gives the same output as **ci2** above.

Figure 9.1 Output for Pearson's correlation in Stata

---

mdi is the mental development index score and *parent* is the parental questionnaire score. Note that we calculate the summary statistics before calculating the correlation.
Select 'Analyze'
Select 'Descriptive Statistics'
Select 'Descriptives'
Move *mdi* and *parent* to 'Variables' box
Select 'Options' and tick boxes for required statistics

Select 'Correlate'
Select 'Bivariate correlations'
Select 'Pearson correlations'
Move *mdi* and *parent* to 'Variables' box

Descriptive Statistics

	N	Minimum	Maximum	Mean	Std. Deviation
mdi	64	50	120	81.37	18.949
parent	64	3	142	69.53	34.997
Valid N (listwise)	64				

Correlations

		mdi	parent
mdi	Pearson Correlation	1	.680
	Sig. (2-tailed)		.000
	N	64	64
parent	Pearson Correlation	.680	1
	Sig. (2-tailed)	.000	
	N	64	64

In the table figures are the repeated about the diagonal

Correlation coefficient

P value

Figure 9.2 Output for Pearson's correlation in SPSS

BOX 9.4 HELPFUL TIPS

Presenting correlation

- Give summary statistics for two variables: number, mean, SD, and possibly range

- Include scatterplot if relationship is unusual or a new finding, where space permits

- Strength of relationship is measured by correlation coefficient itself

- Describe direction and strength of relationship

- The P value only provides evidence that a true relationship exists; it does not measure how strong the relationship is

- In large samples you may obtain a small (weak) correlation which is highly significant. Conversely, in a small sample a strong correlation may have a large P value and not be statistically significant

- Standard statistical packages do not always give a CI for product–moment correlation. A specialist package may be needed

- When variables require transforming to meet the assumptions of correlation, the correlation coefficient *is not back-transformed*

- State which correlation coefficient has been used

- The Pearson product–moment correlation coefficient may be denoted by r

- Spearman's rank correlation may be denoted by ρ (rho)

- Kendall's rank correlation may be denoted by τ (tau)

9.2.3 Calculating and presenting correlations between several variables

Sometimes we wish to investigate the intercorrelation between several variables. We will illustrate this using several measures of baby anthropometry from the birthweight study.

The variables are birthweight, head circumference, upper-arm circumference and crown–heel length. The hypotheses tested, and the assumptions made, are the same as in the previous section (Box 9.2).

Stata and SPSS will produce a compound graph of the individual scatterplots which can be presented if space permits (Fig. 9.3). Figure 9.4 shows the Stata output and Box 9.5 shows how these results can be presented. SPSS output is omitted as it is similar to that shown before.

9.2.4 Comment on results

There are several possible explanations for the differences in strength of relationship between the four measures of baby size. First, they are not all measuring the same thing. All the measures are affected by how mature the baby is at birth and how well grown it is for its gestational age. Birthweight and upper-arm circumference are more affected by the 'fatness' of the baby than are head circumference and crown–heel length.

In addition, birthweight is probably measured with less error than the other measures since its measurement is not affected by the baby moving, unlike crown–heel length. Also, the measurement of upper-arm circumference and head circumference rely on placing a tape around a set part of the body, and so are more prone to measurement error. This illustrates that we always need to interpret the data in the light of what we know, and to try to understand why particular results have occurred.

Note that all the baby anthropometry correlations have very small P values and yet the actual correlations vary in size. This is because the P value is related not only to the size of the correlation, but also to the size of the sample. It is important not to judge the strength of relationship from the P value.

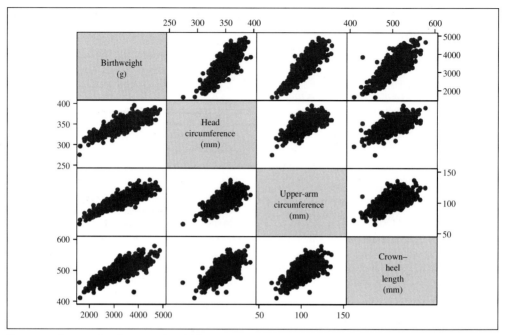

Figure 9.3 Scatterplots for several variables

BOX 9.5 EXAMPLE

Presenting correlations between several variables

Birthweight study

Aim of study To investigate factors related to fetal growth

Study design Cohort study

Patient population Newborn infants whose mothers were booked for delivery at one hospital and from whom detailed baby anthropometry was obtained ($n=198$)

Aim of this analysis To investigate the interrelationship between four measures of baby anthropometry

Description

Table. Correlations (P values) between four measures of anthropometry in 198 newborn infants

	Birthweight	Head circumference	Upper-arm circumference	Crown–heel length
Birthweight	1.00			
Head circumference	0.78 (<0.001)	1.00		
Upper-arm circumference	0.83 (<0.001)	0.63 (<0.001)	1.00	
Crown–heel length	0.79 (<0.001)	0.65 (<0.001)	0.59 (<0.001)	1.00

Methods section

The strength of relationships between birthweight, head circumference, upper-arm circumference, and crown–heel length were estimated using Pearson's correlation coefficient.

Results section

All four measures of baby anthropometry were positively correlated. The strongest linear relationships were between birthweight and the other three measures, ranging between 0.78 and 0.83. Correlations between head circumference, upper-arm length, and crown–heel length were weaker, lying between 0.59 and 0.65.

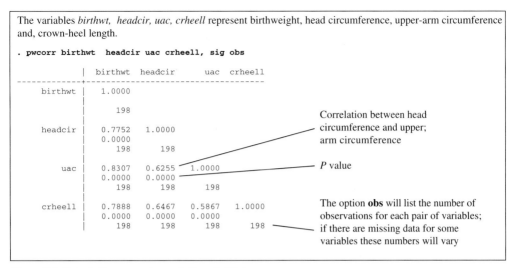

Figure 9.4 Calculating several correlations in Stata

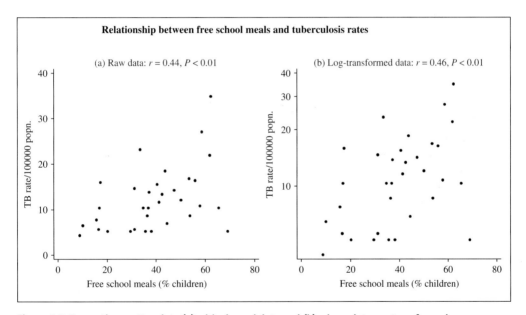

Figure 9.5 Presenting scatterplots (a) with skewed data and (b) where data are transformed

9.2.5 Presenting correlations when data are transformed

The calculation of correlation for transformed data is straightforward as the calculations are performed on the transformed scale and the resulting correlation coefficient is not back-transformed (Box 9.6). However, the presentation of the scatterplot is affected, as we illustrate in Figure 9.5 Hence we will not show the calculation of correlation when variables are transformed but will show the presentation.

Figure 9.5(a) shows a scatterplot of tuberculosis notifications and the percentage of children having free school meals, as an indicator of poverty. These data come from an ecological study conducted in the 33 wards of Liverpool. A correlation of 0.44 ($P < 0.01$) was presented (Spence *et al.* 1993). Tuberculosis rate is skewed and the variability increases as we move from left to right. Therefore the data were log-transformed and the correlation recalculated (Bland and Peacock 2000). Figure 9.5(b) shows the new scatterplot where tuberculosis rate is now given on a logarithmic scale which is equivalent to plotting the transformed data. Tuberculosis rate now follows a reasonably symmetrical distribution. The transformation made little difference to the size of the correlation coefficient, increasing it from 0.44 to 0.46, but that may not always be the case where assumptions are not met.

9.2.6 Rank correlation

If neither of the two variables follows a Normal distribution and transformation is not possible, then a rank correlation can be calculated. To illustrate we will re-do the calculations for the MDI and parental questionnaire data. The distribution of MDI would be expected to be Normal, but in this sample it was slightly irregular, mainly because of several children whose scores were equal to the minimum value possible (50). Therefore we calculate a rank correlation coefficient, Kendall's tau-b, for these data. Spearman's rank correlation could also be used to test the null hypothesis but is less useful as an estimate of the strength of the relationship (see Box 9.7).

9.2.7 Presenting the results for rank correlation

Figure 9.6 shows the Stata output for the calculation of Kendall's tau-b. The corresponding SPSS output is shown in Figure 9.7. The presentation of the rank correlation coefficient is similar to that of Pearson (Box 9.3), but the median and interquartile range can be used as summary measures instead of the mean and standard deviation.

9.2.8 Extending the analysis

Pearson's correlation coefficient can be adjusted to take account of a third variable by calculating the partial correlation coefficient. For example, we could calculate the partial correlation coefficient for the anthropometric data in Box 9.5 after adjusting for gestational age. However, it is usually more informative to use multiple regression to investigate such relationships (see Chapter 10).

9.3 Regression

9.3.1 Introduction

To illustrate linear regression we will use data from a study of health effects of air pollution to estimate the relationship between age and respiratory function in 62 schoolgirls. The scatterplot is shown in Figure 9.8. From this we can see that there is a positive relationship between age and peak flow rate (PEFR). We use regression to estimate how much PEFR increases as age increases. Note that we put the outcome variable (PEFR) on the vertical (y) axis, and the predictor variable (age) on the horizontal (x) axis.

The variables are *mdi* and *parent.*

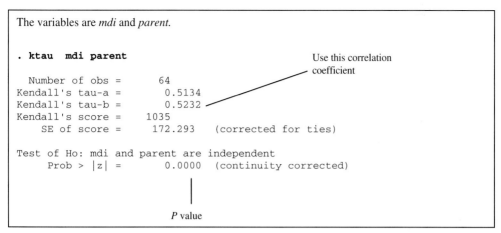

```
.  ktau   mdi parent                              Use this correlation
                                                  coefficient
   Number of obs =        64
Kendall's tau-a =        0.5134
Kendall's tau-b =        0.5232
Kendall's score =      1035
     SE of score =       172.293     (corrected for ties)

Test of Ho: mdi and parent are independent
      Prob > |z| =          0.0000   (continuity corrected)
```

|
P value

Figure 9.6 Output for a rank test in Stata

mdi is the mental development index score and *parent* is the parental questionnaire score. Note that we calculate the summary statistics before calculating the correlation.

Select 'Analyze'
Select 'Correlate'
Select 'Bivariate'
Move *mdi* and *parent* 'Variables' box
Tick 'Kendall's tau-b' box

Correlations

			mdi	parent
Kendall's tau_b	mdi	Correlation Coefficient	1.000	.523
		Sig. (2-tailed)	.	.000
		N	64	64
	parent	Correlation Coefficient	.523	1.000
		Sig. (2-tailed)	.000	.
		N	64	64

Correlation coefficient   P value

Figure 9.7 Output for a rank test in SPSS

Figures 9.9 and 9.10 show the Stata and SPSS outputs. Box 9.8 summaries the key features of linear regression.

9.3.2 Presenting the results of simple linear regression

Box 9.9 shows how to present the results. If space permits, the scatterplot may be given as well. The regression coefficient for age is given with the 95% confidence interval as a measure of precision. Note that summary statistics were presented as well as the regression results to set the findings in context. Box 9.10 gives some helpful tips on presentation.

Since there is only one regression, the findings can easily be presented in the text. If several regressions are done then the results might be better displayed in a table (see section 9.3.3).

The assumptions of Normal residuals and constant variance are not usually reported in a paper or a report. However, in some situations it may be particularly important to justify the analysis, and in such cases the results of testing assumptions should be described in the text.

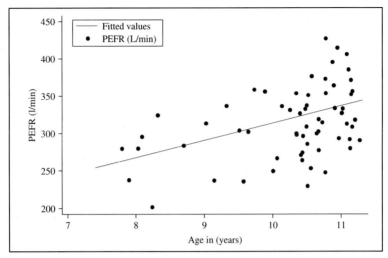

Figure 9.8 Scatterplot of two variables with linear regression line

BOX 9.8 INFORMATION

Regression

Simple linear regression

Null hypothesis There is no linear relationship between the two variables in the population.

Assumptions The distribution of the residuals is Normal. The variance (standard deviation) of the outcome y is constant for different values of the predictor x.

Deviations from assumptions Try transforming the outcome variable.

Checking the assumptions:

- Plot raw data to check for linearity

- Draw histogram or Normal plot of residuals to check that they follow Normal distribution

- May be able to detect heterogeneity of variance from scatterplot. Alternatively, plot residuals against predictor to see if spread of residuals varies across the range of the predictor.

Notes:

- Non-linearity, non-Normality, and non-constant variance sometimes occur together, and so a single transformation may resolve all three deviations

- The P value for the regression coefficient will be the same as the P value for the Pearson correlation coefficient.

BOX 9.10 HELPFUL TIPS

Regression analysis

- Plot the data to investigate the relationship before doing any calculations

- Check that the relationship is reasonably approximated by a straight line

- Check that the assumptions of the regression analysis hold (e.g. Normally distributed residuals). These checks would not usually be reported except perhaps in the text if required.

- Present summary statistics for the data as well as the results of the regression analysis itself

- If the purpose of the analysis is hypothesis testing, then present the regression coefficients and 95% CIs

- If the purpose of the analysis is prediction, then present the equation of the line with standard errors for the coefficients

- If there are several quantitative predictors and/or several outcomes, consider standardising the regression coefficients to make it easier to compare sizes of effects

- When variables require transformation to meet the assumptions of regression, the *interpretation of the regression coefficient is affected by the transformation*

- If there are several possible predictor variables, consider whether there is a need to disentangle their effects and present adjusted effects (see Chapter 10)

pefr and *age* are the outcome and predictor variables. Note that we calculate the summary statistics before doing the regression analysis.

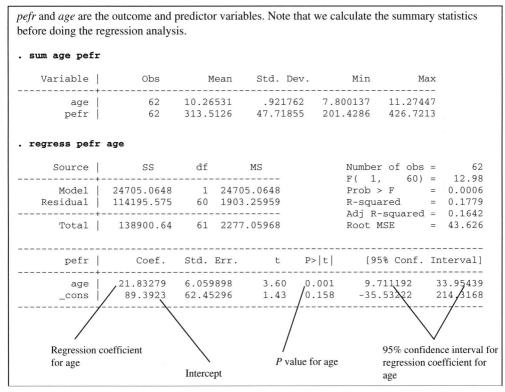

```
. sum age pefr

    Variable |       Obs        Mean    Std. Dev.        Min         Max
-------------+--------------------------------------------------------
         age |        62    10.26531     .921762    7.800137    11.27447
        pefr |        62    313.5126    47.71855    201.4286    426.7213


. regress pefr age

      Source |       SS        df        MS               Number of obs =      62
-------------+------------------------------               F(  1,    60) =   12.98
       Model |  24705.0648      1   24705.0648             Prob > F      =  0.0006
    Residual |  114195.575     60   1903.25959             R-squared     =  0.1779
-------------+------------------------------               Adj R-squared =  0.1642
       Total |   138900.64     61   2277.05968             Root MSE      =  43.626


        pefr |      Coef.   Std. Err.       t     P>|t|      [95% Conf. Interval]
-------------+----------------------------------------------------------------
         age |   21.83279    6.059898     3.60    0.001      9.711192    33.95439
       _cons |    89.3923    62.45296     1.43    0.158     -35.53222     214.3168
```

Regression coefficient for age

Intercept

P value for age

95% confidence interval for regression coefficient for age

Figure 9.9 Output for simple regression in Stata

BOX 9.9 EXAMPLE

Presenting the results for simple regression

Rochester study

Aim of study To investigate effects of air pollution on respiratory function in children.

Study design Cohort study.

Study population Sixty-two primary school age girls.

Aim of analysis To investigate the relationship between peak flow rate and age.

Description

Methods section

The relationship between peak flow rate and age in 62 primary school age girls was estimated using simple linear regression.

Results section

Sixty-two girls aged 7 to 11 years were included in this analysis. Peak flow rate varied from 201 to 427 l/min. There was a significant linear relationship between age and peak flow rate with regression coefficient 21.8 l/min/year (95% CI 9.7 to 34.0), $P = 0.001$.

(Peacock *et al.* 2003)

9.3.3 **Performing and presenting several regressions**

Sometimes we wish to investigate the effects of several factors on an outcome, or investigate the effect of a predictor on several outcomes. To illustrate this we will show some analyses from the birthweight study where the purpose of the analyses was to investigate the effects on mean birthweight of the number of cigarettes smoked and the constituent content of the brand. At the time of the study, tables of the tar, nicotine, and carbon

pefr and *age* are the outcome and predictor variables. Note that we calculate the summary statistics before doing the regression analysis

Descriptive Statistics

	N	Minimum	Maximum	Mean	Std. Deviation
pefr	62	201.4286	426.7213	313.512618	47.7185466
age	62	7.800137	11.274470	10.26530692	.921762187
Valid N (listwise)	62				

Select 'Analyze'
Select 'Regression'
Select 'Linear'
Move *pefr* into the 'Dependent' and *age* into the 'Independent' variables boxes
Select 'Statistics' and tick the 'confidence intervals' box

Variables Entered/Removed(b)

Model	Variables Entered	Variables Removed	Method
1	age(a)	.	Enter

a All requested variables entered.
b Dependent Variable: pefr

ANOVA(b)

Model		Sum of Squares	df	Mean Square	F	Sig.
1	Regression	24705.049	1	24705.049	12.980	.001(a)
	Residual	114195.592	60	1903.260		
	Total	138900.641	61			

a Predictors: (Constant), age
b Dependent Variable: pefr

Coefficients(a)

Model		Unstandardized Coefficients		Standardized Coefficients	t	Sig.	95% Confidence Interval for B	
		B	Std. Error	Beta			Lower Bound	Upper Bound
1	(Constant)	89.392	62.453		1.431	.158	-35.532	214.317
	age	21.833	6.060	.422	3.603	.001	9.711	33.954

a Dependent Variable: pefr

Regression coefficient for age

Intercept

P value for age

Standardised regression coefficient = regression coeff x SD(age)/SD(pefr)

95% confidence interval for regression coefficient for age

From table at top of figure SD(age)=0.9218 and SD(pefr)=47.7185
Standardised regression coefficient
= 21.833x0.9218/47.7185
= 0.422 (see section 9.3.4)

Figure 9.10 Output for simple regression in SPSS

BOX 9.11 EXAMPLE

Presenting the results for several predictor variables

Birthweight study

Aim of study To investigate factors affecting the outcome of pregnancy.

Study design Cohort study.

Study population 457 women who smoked in pregnancy and delivered their baby in one hospital.

Aim of analysis To investigate the effects on birthweight of the number and type of cigarette smoked in pregnancy.

Description

Methods

The relationship between mean birthweight and number smoked, and nicotine, tar, and carbon monoxide content of the brand smoked, were tested using linear regression.

Results

Table A. Summary statistics for birthweight and smoking in 457 pregnant women

Variable	No.	Mean	SD	IQR[1]	Min	Max
Birthweight (g)	457	3204	535	3060–3660	520	4650
Cigs/day	457	10.5	7.5	5–15	1	40
Nicotine (mg/cig)	457	1.28	0.26	1.2–1.4	0.3	1.5
Tar (mg/cig)	457	14.9	3.5	14–17	4	23
Carbon monoxide (mg/cig)	457	15.3	3.7	14–18	3	19

[1] IQR is interquartile range

Table B. Regression coefficients of birthweight on the number of cigarettes smoked, and the nicotine, tar, and carbon monoxide content of the brand smoked, in 457 pregnant women.

Predictor variable	Regression coefficient	95% CI	P value	Standardised coefficient[1]
Cigs/day	−5.3	−11.9, 1.3	0.112	53.3
Nicotine (mg/cig)	−187.5	−377, 2.3	0.053	37.5
Tar (mg/cig)	−16.9	−30.7, −3.1	0.016	50.7
Carbon monoxide (mg/cig)	−17.4	−30.7, −4.2	0.010	69.8

[1] Regression coefficient standardised to an interquartile range change in predictor variable.

There was wide variability in the number of cigarettes smoked, ranging from 1 to 40 per day. Similarly, there was wide variability in constituent content (table A). All four measures of smoke intake were negatively associated with birthweight, but the number of cigarettes was not statistically significant. Of the three measures of smoke content, the standardised regression coefficient suggested that the strongest effect was for carbon monoxide content, and suggested a difference of 70 g in mean birthweight between smokers of low and high carbon monoxide yield cigarettes.

monoxide content of all UK brands were published by the UK Government Chemist.

We will not show the Stata and SPSS outputs as these are similar to those for simple linear regression (Figs 9.9 and 9.10). We will show the presentation of the results and suggest ways to compare regression coefficients for different factors.

Scatterplots (omitted) had shown a negative relationship between birthweight and the number of cigarettes smoked and the constituent content. Box 9.11 shows how the results could be presented, starting with summary statistics.

9.3.4 Standardising regression coefficients

When comparing several regression coefficients, based on variables with different scales, it is useful to standardise them in some way. There are several ways of doing this. In this example, we have expressed the coefficients as the equivalent change in birthweight for a change in predictor across its interquartile range. Box 9.11 shows that the standardised coefficient for cigarettes per day is 53 g. This means that a woman whose cigarette consumption is on the 25th percentile would be expected to have a baby 53 g heavier than a woman whose consumption is on the 75th percentile.

As an alternative, we could have expressed the coefficients in terms of standard deviation changes. If we were comparing coefficients for several outcomes, this means expressing them in terms of the number of standard deviations of the outcome as well as the number of standard deviations of the predictor. This is what SPSS means by its standardised coefficient (Fig. 9.10).

9.3.5 Comment on the results

The analysis showed that several of the variables analysed were associated with the outcome, here birthweight. The next logical step would be to try to disentangle these predictor variables to see if any of their effects could be explained by any of the other variables. This type of analysis requires a multifactorial approach which we will address in Chapter 10.

9.3.6 Log transformations

If the assumptions of regression are not met and the data have to be transformed, then the interpretation of the regression coefficients is changed.

We will give an example to show how this works.

The cellular adhesion molecule concentrations found in the blood of participants of the Wandsworth Heart and Stroke study were skewed and so were log-transformed to give a Normal distribution. An analysis was carried out to examine the relationship between adhesion molecule concentrations and blood pressure. Box 9.12 shows how to calculate the percentage increase in adhesion molecule concentration per 10 mmHg change in blood pressure from the regression analysis. Box 9.13 shows how the analysis can be presented.

9.3.7 Prediction

In the regression examples presented in this section, we have assumed that the main purpose of the regression is hypothesis testing rather than prediction. In such studies we are primarily interested in the slope of the line and the intercept is often not

---

BOX 9.12 EXAMPLE

Back-transforming regression coefficients

Regression coefficient (95% CI) for the relationship between the log transform of sE-selectin (ng/ml) and systolic blood pressure in mmHg was 0.00576 (0.00339 to 0.00813). This was calculated using Stata.

1. Taking exponentials (antilogs) gives 1.005777 (1.003396 to 1.008163).

This is the ratio of the predicted sE-selectin at any blood pressure divided by the predicted sE-selectin 1 mmHg lower.

2. It is more useful to express this as the percentage increase per 1 mmHg change in systolic blood pressure. This is calculated by subtracting 1 and multiplying by 100, i.e. The percentage increase in sE-selectin per unit increase in systolic blood pressure is 0.5777 (95% CI 0.3396 to 0.8163).

3. It may be useful to change the scale because a 1 mm Hg increase in systolic blood pressure is very small and consequently the percentage increase is near to 1. It is more useful to express the increase as per 10 mmHg increase in blood pressure. This can be done by multiplying the regression coefficient by 10 *before* back-transformation, (i.e. $\exp(0.0576) = 1.0593$ giving the percentage increase per 10 mmHg as 5.9.

BOX 9.13 EXAMPLE

Presenting the results of a regression model that uses a log transformation of the predictor variable

Wandsworth Heart and Stroke Study

Aim of study To compare cardiovascular risk factors in three ethnic groups.

Study design Cross-sectional survey with stratified random sampling to obtain equal numbers in each sex–ethnic group category.

Study population 1577 men and women from three ethnic groups living in South London.

Aim of the analysis To examine the relationship between adhesion molecule concentrations and blood pressure.

Presentation

Methods section

Plasma concentration of sE-selectin was positively skewed and therefore analyses were performed on log-transformed data. Linear regression was used to estimate the relationship between adhesion molecules and blood pressure. The regression coefficients were back-transformed and the relationship expressed as percentage change in sE-selectin per 10 mmHg change in blood pressure.

Results section

There was a highly significant positive relationship between systolic blood pressure and sE-selectin in women. A weaker relationship, which was only significant for diastolic blood pressure, was found in men (table).

Table. Relationship between sE-selectin and blood pressure concentrations in men and women

	Men			Women		
	Effect (%)[a]	(95% CI)	P value	Effect (%)[a]	(95% CI)	P value
SBP	1.4	−1.0 to 4.0	0.250	5.9	3.4 to 8.5	<0.001
DBP	4.8	0.5 to 9.3	0.030	11.4	6.5 to 16.5	<0.001

[a] Percentage increase in sE-selectin molecule concentration per 10 mmHg change in blood pressure.
(Miller *et al.* 2004)

reported. If the purpose of the regression is to predict, then the full equation must be reported. Box 9.14 shows the full equation for the relationship between PEFR and age for the study described in Box 9.9. A graph has been included with the confidence interval for the predicted values of PEFR at different ages. Note that the confidence intervals presented in box 9.14 are for the fitted values and not for future predicted values. We would not recommend using these data to predict lung function in another sample as the sample is small and there are few children aged 8–10 years.

If centile charts are to be constructed, it is very important that the regression assumptions were not violated and that the fit to the line is good, so that precise predictions can be made.

9.3.8 Extending the analysis

Where there are several possible predictor variables, it can be useful to look at the effect of one variable after adjusting for the effects of the other variables. In the birthweight analysis we might wish to look at the effect of the number of cigarettes per day, after adjusting for the tar, and carbon monoxide content of the brand. This can be done using multiple regression described in chapter 10.

9.4 Further reading

The references given in Box 9.15 are those that we have found particularly useful for the specific topics listed.

BOX 9.14 EXAMPLE

Presentation of a regression line used for prediction

Rochester study

Aim of study To investigate effects of air pollution on respiratory function in children.

Study design Cohort study.

Study population Sixty-two primary school age girls.

Aim of analysis To investigate the relationship between peak flow rate and age.

Methods section

The relationship between peak flow rate and age in was estimated using simple linear regression.

Results section

Sixty-two girls aged 7 to 11 years were included in this analysis. There was a significant linear relationship between age and peak flow rate with regression coefficient 21.8 l/min/year (95% CI 9.7 to 34.0), $P = 0.001$. The full equation and 95% confidence interval for the predicted values is given in the figure. The expected PEFR increases from 264 l/min at age 8 to 329 l/min at age 11.

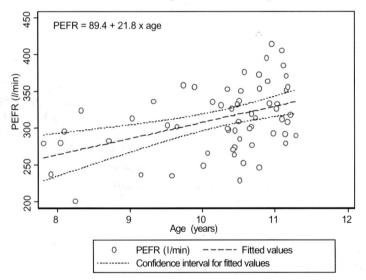

Note: Always label the lines drawn on the graph.

BOX 9.15 **INFORMATION**

Further information on statistical methods

Correlation

Altman (1991, Chapter 11) Armitage *et al.* (2002, Chapter 7) Bland (2000, Chapter 11) Campbell, and Machin (1999, Chapter 7) Kirkwood and Sterne (2003, Chapter 10)

Regression

Altman (1991, Chapter 11) Armitage *et al.* (2002, Chapter 7) Bland (2000, Chapter 11), Campbell and Machin (1999, Chapter 7), Kirkwood and Sterne (2003, Chapter 10)

Chapter summary

Analysing relationships between variables

- Always plot the data before doing any analysis
- Present summary statistics for the variables analysed
- In the methods section, describe the method clearly, distinguishing between:

  *regression and correlation
  *product moment correlation and rank correlation

- In the results section, distinguish between:

  *regression coefficient and correlation coefficient
  *coefficient value and P value (strength of relationship is measured by the coefficient not by P value)
  *positive and negative relationships

- For correlation give coefficient, P value, and number of subjects (and possibly 95% CI)
- For regression, present coefficient, 95% CI, P value, and number of subjects
- Report any transformations of the data
- Check that the assumptions of the method hold, although this is not usually reported in papers and reports

CHAPTER 10

Multifactorial analyses

10.1 Introduction

In this chapter we will look at how to present one-way analysis of variance, multiple regression, and logistic regression analyses. One-way analysis of variance is an extension of the two-sample t test (Chapter 7) and is used to compare more than two independent groups. Multiple regression is used when we have a continuous outcome variable and several possible predictor variables and is an extension of simple linear regression (Chapter 9) or analysis of variance. Note that the terms 'predictor variables', 'explanatory variables', and 'independent variables' are used interchangeably.

In this book two-way analysis of variance has been treated as multiple regression (section 10.3.4) but we have not covered interaction terms in detail. Analysis of covariance where we wish to investigate the effect of a categorical variable adjusting for the effect of a continuous confounder is again covered under multiple regression (section 10.3.1).

Logistic regression is used when we have a binary outcome and several possible predictor variables and is an extension of the chi-squared method (Chapter 7) and odds ratios. Box 10.1 summarises when to use each of these methods.

10.1.1 Planning the analysis

Any complex dataset could give rise to a multitude of statistical comparisons, all with a 5% chance of spurious statistical significance. Before carrying out any multifactorial analysis it is useful to identify the purpose of the analysis, decide which comparisons are of primary interest, and draw up a plan of analysis (section 3.7). These may have been done when the study was designed, but sometimes research questions are identified after the protocol was written. A clear plan will help one to avoid being overwhelmed by output from the computer, will simplify the reporting of the results, and will help to avoid spurious significant findings.

10.1.2 Preliminary presentation of the data

Before beginning to present complex analyses, the sample should be described as in section 5.7, and

summary statistics should be reported for the key variables. It is usually helpful to perform and describe basic unifactorial analyses prior to doing multifactorial analysis. The summary statistics should be appropriate for the multifactorial analysis. For example, means, differences in means, and slopes could all be described prior to multiple regression, while medians and ranges would be less relevant. Since rank methods are usually used where there are problems in fulfilling the Normality assumptions, it would be illogical to follow a unifactorial analysis using rank tests with a multiple regression analysis.

When using logistic regression to adjust for confounders, it is preferable to describe the unifactorial relationships in terms of odds ratios, even though in some circumstances relative risk would be equally valid. The unifactorial and multifactorial associations are then directly comparable.

To avoid repetition, we have not in general included a description of either the sample or the unifactorial analyses in the examples of presentation given in this chapter. Many examples of presenting these basic descriptive data are given throughout the earlier chapters. However, we have assumed that in any publication or report, unifactorial analyses will be described as far as space permits so as to give the reader a better understanding of the data.

10.1.3 Missing data

As far as possible, steps should be taken to avoid missing data, but in medical and health care research some missing data are inevitable. This can cause problems in the presentation and analysis of the data.

In multifactorial analysis we can either use all the available data in any analysis or restrict our analysis to only those subjects with complete data for the variables we wish to include. Which we choose depends on how many missing cases there are, and is a matter of judgement.

The data shown in Box 5.5 illustrate some of the issues that arise when reporting analyses where there are missing data. First, the table shown gives both unadjusted and age-adjusted relative risks for all predictor variables. Since age was available for all subjects, these two relative risks were calculated using the same set of subjects. Secondly, in this study there were some missing data for the other predictor variables; for example ethnic origin was only available for 1096/1201 subjects, and social class only was available for 1036/1201.

In order to make maximum use of the data, the analyses used all observations available for each predictor variable. To make this clear, the table shows the total number of observations for each of these, and gives the numbers with the various characteristics. The consequence of using all observations available for each predictor variable is that the relative risks for the different variables are calculated using slightly different sets of subjects.

If the number of missing observations is minimal, then it may be easier to produce a subset of subjects with complete data. If this is done, it should be explained in the methods section. The advantage is that all the analysis is carried out on the same subjects, and any differences between adjusted and unadjusted results are due to the variables adjusted for and not the subset of subjects analysed. The presentation is simpler as we only need to state the number of subjects once.

In this chapter we have used datasets where all variables are complete and the number of subjects is constant regardless of which variables are being included in the regression models (see Figs. 10.3 and 10.4).

10.2 **One-way analysis of variance**

10.2.1 **Introduction**

One-way analysis of variance is used to compare the means of a continuous variable from more than two groups. Once it has been shown that there is a significant difference between the groups, it is often of interest to compare particular groups with each other. Care needs to be taken at this point, since if there are several groups, there will be many possible comparisons that could be made. In order to preserve the overall P value and avoid spurious significant results, the number of comparisons can be reduced by deciding in advance which subgroups are really of interest and then using a method which adjusts the P value to allow for the number of comparisons made (see Box 10.2).

> **BOX 10.2 INFORMATION**
>
> ## One-way analysis of variance
>
> *Null hypothesis* The groups all come from populations with the same mean
>
> *Assumptions*
>
> - Data are continuous
> - Data follow a Normal distribution within each group
> - Standard deviations in the groups are the same
>
> *Deviations from assumptions*
>
> - Try transformation
> - If data are positively skewed and the SD increases with the mean, then log transformation will often correct these two problems
>
> *Checking the assumptions*
>
> - Look at distribution of residuals (observed value minus group mean)
>
> *Multiple comparisons*
>
> - If the overall P value for the group is significant, then pairs of groups may be tested. Do not test pairs of groups if the overall P value is greater than 0.05 (or the chosen level of significance).
> - Only test comparisons that you are really interested in
> - Use a method which preserves the overall P value to avoid spurious significant results in subgroups (e.g. Scheffé, Bonferroni, Newman–Keuls, Duncan)
> - For further reading see Box 10.16
>
> *Note* If there are only two groups, then the P value from analysis of variance will be the same as that from the t test

In this section we will use data from the birthweight study and will analyse the effects of smoking in early pregnancy on mean birthweight. Women are categorised into five groups: never smokers, quitters before pregnancy, quitters in early pregnancy, smoke 1–14 cigarettes/day, and smoke 15+ cigarettes/day. To do this analysis, we first calculated summary statistics for the five groups and then did the one-way analysis of variance. Multiple comparisons of pairs of groups were performed using Scheffé's test to investigate the effects of quitting smoking at different stages. Figures 10.1 and 10.2 show the Stata and SPSS outputs.

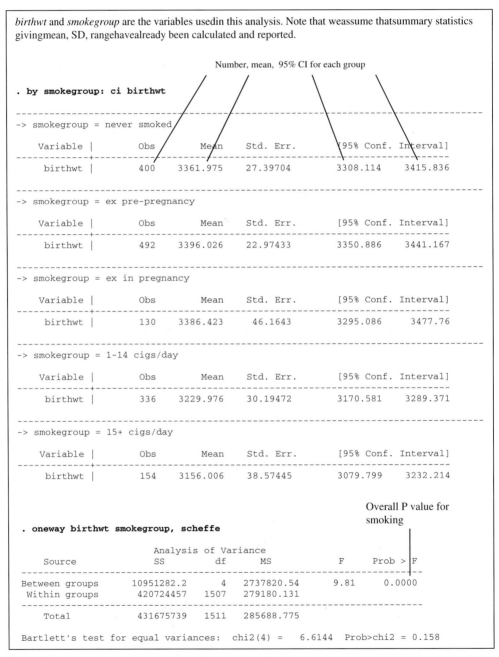

Figure 10.1 Output for one-way analysis of variance in Stata

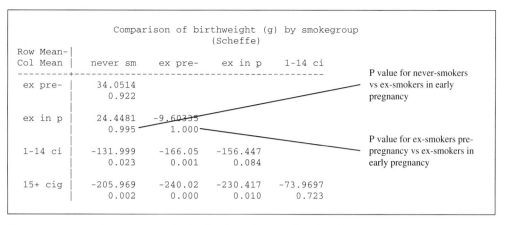

Figure 10.1 Output for one-way analysis of variance in Stata (continued)

birthwt and*smokegroup* are the variables used in this analysis.
Select 'Analyze'
Select 'Compare means'
Select 'One-way ANOVA'
Move*birthwt*into'Dependent List' box and *smokegroup* to 'Factor' box
Select 'Options' and then 'Descriptive'
Select'Post Hoc' and thentick 'Scheffé'

Descriptives

birthwt

	N	Mean	Std. Deviation	Std. Error	95% Confidence Interval for Mean		Minimum	Maximum
					Lower Bound	Upper Bound		
never smoked	400	3361.98	547.941	27.397	3308.11	3415.84	960	4870
ex pre-pregnancy	492	3396.03	509.595	22.974	3350.89	3441.17	1160	4760
ex in pregnancy	130	3386.42	526.354	46.164	3295.09	3477.76	1140	4720
1-14 cigs/day	336	3229.98	553.478	30.195	3170.58	3289.37	520	4650
15+ cigs/day	154	3156.01	478.696	38.574	3079.80	3232.21	1330	4420
Total	1512	3324.85	534.499	13.746	3297.88	3351.81	520	4870

Number, mean, 95% CI for each group

ANOVA

birthwt

	Sum of Squares	df	Mean Square	F	Sig.
Between Groups	10951282.154	4	2737820.539	9.807	.000
Within Groups	420724456.940	1507	279180.131		
Total	431675739.095	1511			

Overall *P* value for smoking

Figure 10.2 Output for one-way analysis of variance in SPSS

Multiple Comparisons

P value for never-smokers vs exsmokers in pre-pregnancy

Dependent Variable: birthwt
Scheffe

(I) smokegroup	(J) smokegroup	Mean Difference (I-J)	Std. Error	Sig.	95% Confidence Interval	
					Lower Bound	Upper Bound
never smoked	ex pre-pregnancy	-34.051	35.572	.922	-143.76	75.66
	ex in pregnancy	-24.448	53.343	.995	-188.96	140.06
	1-14 cigs/day	131.999(*)	39.100	.023	11.41	252.59
	15+ cigs/day	205.969(*)	50.108	.002	51.43	360.50
ex pre-pregnancy	never smoked	34.051	35.572	.922	-75.66	143.76
	ex in pregnancy	9.603	52.105	1.000	-151.09	170.30
	1-14 cigs/day	166.050(*)	37.394	.001	50.72	281.38
	15+ cigs/day	240.020(*)	48.788	.000	89.55	390.49
ex in pregnancy	never smoked	24.448	53.343	.995	-140.06	188.96
	ex pre-pregnancy	-9.603	52.105	1.000	-170.30	151.09
	1-14 cigs/day	156.447	54.575	.084	-11.86	324.76
	15+ cigs/day	230.417(*)	62.932	.010	36.33	424.50
1-14 cigs/day	never smoked	-131.999(*)	39.100	.023	-252.59	-11.41
	ex pre-pregnancy	-166.050(*)	37.394	.001	-281.38	-50.72
	ex in pregnancy	-156.447	54.575	.084	-324.76	11.86
	15+ cigs/day	73.970	51.417	.723	-84.60	232.54
15+ cigs/day	never smoked	-205.969(*)	50.108	.002	-360.50	-51.43
	ex pre-pregnancy	-240.020(*)	48.788	.000	-390.49	-89.55
	ex in pregnancy	-230.417(*)	62.932	.010	-424.50	-36.33
	1-14 cigs/day	-73.970	51.417	.723	-232.54	84.60

* The mean difference is significant at the .05 level.

All comparisons are given twice in this table with the difference in means having opposite signs. The difference is the category in the first column minus the category in the second column. The *P* value is the same.

Difference in mean birthweight between 15+ cigs/day and 1-14 cigs/day and 95% CI

Figure 10.2 Output for one-way analysis of variance in SPSS (continued)

10.2.2 Presenting the results of one-way analysis of variance

Box 10.3 shows how to present the results of one-way analysis of variance. The mean values for the different groups are shown with 95% confidence intervals and the overall *P* value for comparing the groups. Since this *P* value was very small (<0.0001), it was reasonable to compare pairs of groups, specifically the ex-smokers. If the overall variability is not significant, pairwise comparisons should not be done.

BOX 10.3 EXAMPLE

Presenting the results for one-way analysis of variance

Birthweight study

Aim of study To investigate effects of smoking on outcome of pregnancy.

Study design Cohort study

Study population 1512 pregnant women delivering at one hospital.

Aim of analysis To investigate the effects of smoking on birthweight and to see if quitting affected mean birthweight.

Description

Methods section

The differences in mean birthweight in never smokers, smokers quitting before pregnancy, smokers quitting in early pregnancy, light smokers (1–14 per day), and heavy smokers (15+ per day) were tested using one-way analysis of variance. Multiple comparison were performed using Scheffés test.

Results section

Table. Mean birthweight by smoking in early pregnancy

Smoking group	No.	Mean birthweight (g)	95%CI	P value
Never smoker	400	3362	3308, 3416	<0.0001
Quit before pregnancy	492	3396	3351, 3441	
Quit in early pregnancy	130	3386	3295, 3478	
1–14 cigs/day	336	3230	3171, 3289	
15+cigs/day	154	3156	3080, 3232	

Thirty-two per cent of women (490/1512) reported smoking in early pregnancy. There was highly significant variation between mean birthweight in the five groups. The babies of heavy smokers weighed on average 206 g less than babies of never smokers ($P = 0.002$). Women who quit smoking in early pregnancy had a very similar mean birthweight to women who never smoked (difference=24 g, $P > 0.99$). There was no evidence for any difference in mean birthweight in women who had quit before pregnancy compared with those who quit in early pregnancy (difference=10 g, $P > 0.99$) (table).

10.2.3 Reference categories

In Box 10.3, the means are presented with their 95% confidence intervals, and comparisons between categories are given in the text. An alternative presentation would be to treat one category as the 'reference' and to present the differences and their 95% confidence intervals in the table, as has been done for alcohol consumption in Box 10.8. Figure 10.2 shows all the differences and their 95% confidence intervals, which are produced by default in SPSS for the different smoking categories. For Stata, the method shown in Figure 10.7 can be used.

In some situations there is no obvious reference category and giving the means for each group is preferable, as in Box 10.3. Reference categories are discussed further in section 10.3.3.

10.2.4 Further analyses

With smoking data, it may be reasonable to look for evidence of a dose–response effect. In these data, the never-smokers and the two ex-smoking groups were not significantly different, and so these could be combined to form three groups: non-smokers, light smokers, and heavy smokers. A linear trend in these could be tested to investigate dose–response. There are several ways that this could be done, but one way would be to fit a simple linear regression through the groups, coding them 1, 2, and 3, and looking at the overall P value. This gives $P<0.001$, suggesting that there is some evidence for a dose–response relationship.

10.2.5 Kruskal–Wallis analysis of variance

This is an extension of the Mann–Whitney U test to compare three or more groups and has similar properties to the Mann–Whitney test (see Box 7.5). As described in the previous section, an overall P value should be calculated and presented first, but medians and ranges are more suitable as summary statistics as for the Mann–Whitney U test.

10.3 Multiple regression

10.3.1 Introduction

Often we have a continuous outcome variable and several predictor variables and we want to see the effects of one or more of these after adjusting for confounding variables. In Chapter 9 we showed that lung function was related to age in the Rochester study (section 9.3.1). We now want to investigate gas cooking in the home and see if it is related to PEFR after allowing for other possible confounders such as wheeziness, parental smoking, and age. We can do this using multiple regression analysis. Box 10.4 summarises the main features of multiple regression analysis.

The Stata and SPSS outputs are shown in Figures 10.3 and 10.4. In the Stata output the first model fitted all four predictor variables and showed that *smokers* and *wheeze* were non-significant ($P=0.839$ $P=0.100$, respectively). Since *smokers* had the larger P value of the two, it was removed from the model and the regression was repeated without it. This regression showed that *wheeze* remained non-significant ($P=0.099$), and so *wheeze* was removed and the model was fitted with just *age* and *gas* (cooking). Both of these variables remained significant and so this was the final model reported.

The SPSS output is reduced so that only the first model and final model results are displayed to reduce repetition and save space.

10.3.2 Presenting multiple regression analyses

Box 10.5 shows how to present the results. We have assumed that summary statistics would have been calculated and already presented as described in

---

> **BOX 10.4 INFORMATION**
>
> ### Multiple regression
>
> *Null hypothesis* There is no linear relationship between the outcome and the predictor variable.
>
> *Note* This hypothesis applies separately to each predictor variable in the model.
>
> *Use for*
> - Continuous outcome and several predictor variables
> - Predictors can be continuous, binary, or categorical (see note below)
>
> *Assumptions* The distribution of the residuals is Normal. The variance of the outcome y is constant for different values of each predictor x.
>
> *Deviations from assumptions:*
> - Try transforming the outcome variable
> - If the relationship is not linear, then either a transformation may be used to model the actual relationship, or the variable may be categorised into several groups
>
> *Checking the assumptions:*
> - Plot raw data to check for linearity
> - Draw histogram or Normal plot of residuals to check they follow Normal distribution
> - May be able to detect heterogeneity of variance from scatterplot. Alternatively, plot residuals against predictor to see if spread of residuals varies across the range of the predictor
>
> *Cautionary note on categorical variables with more than two groups*
> Care needs to be taken that these are not treated as continuous variables within a statistical package.
>
> Section 10.3.3 shows how this can be done in Stata and SPSS.

Chapter 5. The results of unifactorial analyses of possible predictor variables may be presented if space permits. This would be presented in a similar way to the unifactorial analyses shown in Chapters 7 and 9.

The direction of the difference for the binary predictor variables can be deduced from the

pefr, age, gas, smokers, wheeze are the variables used in this analysis. Note that the first regression includes all the variables, whereas the second only includes those that were significant in the first. The variables *gas, smokers, wheeze* are all coded 1=yes, 0=no, hence the regression coefficient is the difference in mean PEFR between those exposed and those not exposed.

Smoking is non-significant and has the largest *P* value (=0.839). Remove this variable and repeat regression.

. **regress pefr   age   gas smokers wheeze**

Source	SS	df	MS
Model	39918.5953	4	9979.64883
Residual	97152.6004	56	1734.86786
Total	137071.196	60	2284.51993

Number of obs =	61
F(4, 56) =	5.75
Prob > F =	0.0006
R-squared =	0.2912
Adj R-squared =	0.2406
Root MSE =	41.652

pefr	Coef.	Std. Err.	t	P>|t|	[95% Conf. Interval]	
age	24.74714	5.867251	4.22	0.000	12.99363	36.50066
gas	-22.72422	10.97092	-2.07	0.043	-44.70161	-.7468293
smokers	2.216041	10.86123	0.20	0.839	-19.54161	23.97369
wheeze	-24.01984	14.37023	-1.67	0.100	-52.80686	4.767176
_cons	75.4658	60.13859	1.25	0.215	-45.00627	195.9379

. **regress   pefr age gas wheeze**   (note the ANOVA table has been omitted due to lack of space)

Wheeze is non-significant (*P*=0.099) so remove this variable and repeat regression.

pefr	Coef.	Std. Err.	t	P>|t|	[95% Conf. Interval]	
age	24.70649	5.814361	4.25	0.000	13.06343	36.34954
gas	-22.74017	10.87802	-2.09	0.041	-44.52304	-.9573128
wheeze	-23.52698	14.04615	-1.67	0.099	-51.65391	4.599944
_cons	76.81974	59.26674	1.30	0.200	-41.85986	195.4993

. **regress pefr   age   gas**

Source	SS	df	MS
Model	35060.9519	2	17530.4759
Residual	102010.244	58	1758.79731
Total	137071.196	60	2284.51993

Number of obs =	61
F(2, 58) =	9.97
Prob > F =	0.0002
R-squared =	0.2558
Adj R-squared =	0.2301
Root MSE =	41.938

pefr	Coef.	Std. Err.	t	P>|t|	[95% Conf. Interval]	
age	24.01191	5.889133	4.08	0.000	12.22353	35.80029
gas	-26.00182	10.86762	-2.39	0.020	-47.75571	-4.247918
_cons	29.41294	64.96578	0.45	0.652	-100.6302	159.4561

Coefficient, 95% CI, *P* value for age in this row

Coefficient, 95% CI, *P* value for gas cooking in this row

Notes:
1. The constant term, indicated by_cons, is usually left in the model whether it is significant or not
2. There were no missing data for any variables analysed here

Figure 10.3 Output for multiple regression in Stata

pefr, age, gas, smokers, wheeze are the variables used in this analysis. The variables *gas, smokers, wheeze* are all coded 1=yes, 0=no; hence the regression coefficient is the difference in mean PEFR between those exposed and those not exposed.

Select 'Analyze'
Select 'Regression'
Select 'Linear'
Move *pefr* into the 'Dependent' and *age, gas , smokers* and *wheeze* into the 'Independent' variables boxes Select 'Statistics' and tick the 'Confidence Intervals' box

Variables Entered/Removed (b)

Table not shown

Model Summary

Model	R	R Square	Adjusted R Square	Std. Error of the Estimate
1	.540(a)	.291	.241	41.6517434

a Predictors: (Constant), wheeze, age, smokers, gas

ANOVA(b)

Model		Sum of Squares	df	Mean Square	F	Sig.
1	Regression	39918.599	4	9979.650	5.752	.001(a)
	Residual	97152.593	56	1734.868		
	Total	137071.192	60			

a Predictors: (Constant), wheeze, age, smokers, gas
b Dependent Variable: pefr

Coefficients(a)

Model		Unstandardized Coefficients		Standardized Coefficients	t	Sig.	95% Confidence Interval for B	
		B	Std. Error	Beta			Lower Bound	Upper Bound
1	(Constant)	75.466	60.139		1.255	.215	-45.006	195.938
	age	24.747	5.867	.481	4.218	.000	12.994	36.501
	gas	-22.724	10.971	-.239	-2.071	.043	-44.702	-.747
	smokers	2.216	10.861	.023	.204	.839	-19.542	23.974
	wheeze	-24.020	14.370	-.195	-1.672	.100	-52.807	4.767

a Dependent Variable: pefr

For explanation of standardised coefficients see Figure 9.10

P values for parental smoking and wheeze were not significant. Smoking had the largest *P* value and so was removed and regression repeated with age, gas, wheeze (not shown). This showed that wheeze was not significant (*P*=0.099) and so it was removed and regression repeated with age and gas only.

Coefficients(a)

Model		Unstandardized Coefficients		Standardized Coefficients	t	Sig.	95% Confidence Interval for B	
		B	Std. Error	Beta			Lower Bound	Upper Bound
1	(Constant)	81.417	60.118		1.354	.181	-38.922	201.755
	age	24.012	5.889	.467	4.077	.000	12.224	35.800
	gas	-26.002	10.868	-.274	-2.393	.020	4 7.756	-4.248

a Dependent Variable: pefr

Coefficient, 95%CI, *P* value for age in this row
Coefficient, 95% CI, *P* value for gas cooking in this row

Figure 10.4 Output for multiple regression in SPSS

BOX 10.5 EXAMPLE

Presenting the results of multiple regression

Rochester study

Aim of study To investigate effects of air pollution on respiratory function in children.

Study design: Cross-sectional study.

Study population: Sixty-one primary school age girls.

Aim of analysis To see if there was any relationship between gas cooking at home and peak flow rate after allowing for confounding variables.

Description

Methods section

The relationship between peak flow rate and gas cooking was estimated using multiple regression allowing for parental smoking, current wheeze, and age. Non-significant variables were removed one by one, removing the largest P value first, until all remaining variables in the model were significant.

Results section

Table. Multiple regression of peak flow rate (L/min) on gas cooking and age in 61 primary school girls

Variable	Coefficient	95% CI	P value
Gas cooking (yes−no)	−26.0	−47.8, −4.2	0.02
Age (years)	24.0	12.2, 35.8	<0.0001

When the four predictor variables were modelled together, there was no significant effect of parental smoking (coefficient 2.2, [95%CI −19.5,24.0], P=0.84) or current wheeze (−24.0, [−52.8, 4.8], P=0.10). When smoking was removed from the model, the effect of wheeze was similar in size and still non-significant, and age and gas cooking remained significant. Girls who were exposed to gas cooking had a reduction in PEFR of 26 L/min (95%CI [4, 48]) after adjusting for age (table).

Discussion points

Although the effect of current wheeze was not significant, the effect size was similar to that for gas cooking. It is likely that any effect of wheeze is confounded by treatment, which was not recorded.

---

coding and is made clear in the table in Box 10.5. In Stata and SPSS, the coefficient is the difference in mean outcome between the level with the highest code (here 1) and the lowest code (here 0). Box 10.6 gives tips on interpreting regression coefficients.

We have not included a table for the first analysis of all four predictor variables, but have reported the results of this in the text. It is informative to report these results to give a full picture of the analysis that was done, although if many variables were tested, there may not be sufficient space in a paper. We can see that although current wheeze was not significantly related to PEFR, the size of the effect was similar to that of gas cooking.

In general, it is important to describe any non-significant findings as well as any significant ones, because non-significance may simply be due to small sample size and there might indeed be a real effect. By presenting these data and discussing the size of the effect and the possible reasons for non-significance, the researcher allows readers to draw their own conclusions in the light of this and other evidence.

As with simple linear regression, the testing of assumptions is not usually reported in the text.

10.3.3 Presenting multiple regression with categorical variables

In multiple regression we can have continuous or categorical predictor variables, or a mixture of the two. As we have already shown, categorical predictor

BOX 10.6 **HELPFUL TIPS**

Multiple regression: interpreting the coefficients

Continuous predictor variables

- Slope or gradient of the line, i.e. change in outcome for a unit change in predictor

Binary predictor variables

- Difference in mean outcome between the two binary outcomes. For example, if the variable is smoking, then we obtain the difference in mean outcome between smokers and non-smokers.

- It is important to know the coding for the variable under consideration to be able to determine which direction the difference is in

- If the variable is coded 0=no, 1=yes, then in Stata and SPSS, the difference will be the mean outcome (yes – no)

Categorical predictor variables:

- Difference in mean outcome between given category and reference category

- Stata uses different reference categories according to the procedure used (Box 10.7), while SPSS allows lowest code or highest code to be chosen

BOX 10.7 **HELPFUL TIPS**

Categorical variables with more than two groups in multiple regression using Stata and SPSS

Stata

- Can use either **xi:regress** (Fig. 10.5) or **anova** (Fig. 10.7)

- **xi:regress** uses the lowest category as the reference

- **anova** uses the highest category as the reference

- use **anova** if interaction terms are required (see section 10.3.4)

- **anova** will assume variables are categorical unless specified otherwise (see Fig. 10.7)

SPSS

- Use **General Linear Model** not **linear regression**

- Can choose reference category to be first or last

- Interactions will be fitted by default (see section 10.3.4 and Fig. 10.6)

Both programs

- The reference category should not contain a small number of observations, otherwise comparisons with it will be imprecise

- The reference category should be one that aids interpretation; for example, it is more reasonable to choose non-drinkers than heavy drinkers as a reference category

variables with two categories (binary variables) are presented in the same way as continuous predictor variables. When the predictor variable has more than two categories, the presentation is slightly different. In the birthweight study, alcohol intake was divided into five categories and smokers were divided into light and heavy smokers. Figures 10.5 and 10.6 show the results of a multiple regression analysis to investigate the effects of alcohol intake and heavy smoking among the 457 women who smoked. This analysis arose from the observation that alcohol consumption was associated with reduced birthweight in smokers, and so this analysis included smoking and alcohol intake to try to disentangle the effects.

Not only is the presentation different when there are more than two categories, but the computation also involves different procedures. In Stata the command **xi:regress** is used instead of **regress** and in

SPSS the General Linear Model procedure needs to be used, otherwise the categorical variable will be treated as continuous (Box 10.7).

Box 10.8 shows how to present the results. As before, we have assumed that summary statistics have already been presented. We have shown the regression coefficients and 95% confidence intervals. When we have categorical predictor variables, a coefficient is not calculated for each category but instead one category is used as the reference and all other categories are compared with it. It is important to state what the reference category is to aid interpretation of the results.

BOX 10.8 EXAMPLE

Presentation of multiple regression with categorical predictor variables

Birthweight study

Aim of study To investigate effects of smoking on outcome of pregnancy.

Study design Cohort study.

Study population 457 women who smoked in pregnancy and delivered their baby at one hospital.

Aim of analysis To investigate the effects of smoking and alcohol on birthweight for gestational age, expressed as a ratio.

Description

Methods section

The relationship between standardised birthweight ratio, smoking, and alcohol intake in pregnancy was estimated using multiple regression. The results are presented as regression coefficients and 95% confidence intervals.

Results section

Table. Effects of smoking and alcohol intake in pregnancy on birthweight for gestational age in 457 women

Variable	Coefficient	95% CI	Overall P value
Smoking[1]			
Heavy smoking	−0.06	−0.08, −0.03	<0.0001
Alcohol[2] (g/week)			
1–19	−0.02	−0.05, 0.01	0.008
20–49	−0.04	−0.07, −0.01	
50–99	−0.06	−0.11, −0.01	
100+	−0.07	−0.13, −0.02	

[1]Compared with light smokers (reference category).

[2]Compared with non-drinkers (reference category).

There was a significant reduction in mean adjusted birthweight in heavy smokers compared with light smokers after allowing for alcohol intake. Similarly, there was a significant overall effect of alcohol on birthweight for gestational age after allowing for smoking. Mean birthweight decreased steadily as alcohol intake increased.

(Peacock *et al.* 1991).

The choice of reference category is usually made by the statistical program (Box 10.7). By recoding a variable, it is possible to make another level the reference. This might be necessary if the default level contains very few observations and so every comparison would be imprecisely estimated.

Note that we do not present the individual P values for the different levels of the predictor variable, but instead give just the overall P value. Individual levels of the variable may not be statistically significantly different from the reference category, possibly because of small numbers, but that is not a major concern. We are really interested in knowing if there is an overall effect of alcohol.

10.3.4 Multiple regression or analysis of variance?

Analysis of variance estimates the amount of the total variability in a continuous outcome which can be explained by each explanatory variable or group of explanatory variables. These explanatory variables can be continuous or categorical. Analysis of variance tables are often displayed for regression

The variables are slightly different from Figures 10.1 and 10.2.

cigsgp is the grouping variable for smoking and has two categories, light smokers and heavy smokers. These were coded 1, 2 respectively

alcgroup represents five categories of alcohol intake range 0, 1–19, 20–49, 50–99, 100+ g per week. These were coded 0, 1, 2, 3, 4

adjbw is the outcome and represents standardised birthweight as a ratio (birthweight for gestational age)
Further details of these variables are omitted but can be found in Peacock et al. (1991).

```
. xi: regress adjbw  i.cigsgp i.alcgroup
i.cigsgp           _Icigsgp_1-2        (naturally coded; _Icigsgp_1 omitted)
i.alcgroup         _Ialcgroup_0-4      (naturally coded; _Ialcgroup_0 omitted)

      Source |       SS       df       MS              Number of obs =     456
-------------+------------------------------           F(  5,    450) =    5.48
       Model |  .416319047     5  .083263809           Prob > F      =  0.0001
    Residual |  6.84185173    450  .015204115           R-squared     =  0.0574
-------------+------------------------------           Adj R-squared =  0.0469
       Total |  7.25817077    455  .015952024           Root MSE      =  .1233


       adjbw |     Coef.   Std. Err.      t    P>|t|     [95% Conf. Interval]
-------------+----------------------------------------------------------------
  _Icigsgp_2 |  -.0553906   .0147751    -3.75   0.000    -.0844274   -.0263538
 _Ialcgroup_1 |  -.0168603   .0145368    -1.16   0.247    -.0454287    .0117081
 _Ialcgroup_2 |  -.0382412   .0155193    -2.46   0.014    -.0687405   -.0077419
 _Ialcgroup_3 |  -.0577793   .0245754    -2.35   0.019    -.1060762   -.0094825
 _Ialcgroup_4 |  -.0742407   .028292     -2.62   0.009    -.1298416   -.0186398
       _cons |   1.068829   .0150422    71.06   0.000     1.039268    1.098391


. test  _Ialcgroup_1 _Ialcgroup_2 _Ialcgroup_3 _Ialcgroup_4

 ( 1)  _Ialcgroup_1 = 0
 ( 2)  _Ialcgroup_2 = 0
 ( 3)  _Ialcgroup_3 = 0
 ( 4)  _Ialcgroup_4 = 0

       F(  4,    450) =    3.53
            Prob > F =    0.0075
```

P value for smoking

Coefficient for heavy smoking vs light smoking (light smoking is reference category)

Overall *P* value for alcohol

Coefficient for 1–19 g/week alcohol vs non-drinkers (non-drinker is reference category)

Figure 10.5 Output from multiple regression with categorical predictor variables in Stata using xi:regress

models as in Figures 9.9, 9.10, 10.3, and 10.4. If only one explanatory variable is used, then the *P* values from the analysis of variance and the regression analysis will be the same.

Provided that the variables are correctly specified, analysis of variance and multiple regression will do exactly the same calculations. In Stata it is possible to carry out the same analysis and obtain the same results as in Figure 10.5 using the **anova** command. This is shown in Figure 10.7.

Analysis of variance will treat each variable as a whole and give an overall *P* value, while regression

The variables are slightly different from Figures 10.1 and 10.2.

cigsgp is the grouping variable for smoking and has two categories, light smokers and heavy smokers. These were coded 1, 2 respectively

alcgroup represents five categories of alcohol intake ranging, 0, 1–19, 20–49, 50–99, 100+g per week. These were coded 0,1,2,3,4

adjbw is the outcome and represents a standardised birthweight score (birthweight for gestational age)

 Further details of these variables are omitted but can be found in Peacock et al. (1991).

Select 'Analyze'

Select 'General Linear Model'

Select 'Univariate'

Move *adjbwt* to 'Dependent variable' List

Move *alcgroup* and *cigsgrp* to 'Fixed Factors' List

Select 'Model'

Select 'Custom' (Note; the default model is to fit all the interaction terms)

Move *alcgroup* and *cigsgrp* to 'Model' box

Select 'Contrasts'

For each variable highlight the variable and then select 'Simple' from the contrast list and 'first' as the reference category. Click 'Change'

 Note: If a continuous variable were to be added to the model then these are added as 'covariates'

Between-Subjects Factors

Table not shown

Tests of Between-Subjects Effects

Dependent Variable: adjbw

Source	Type III Sum of Squares	df	Mean Square	F	Sig.
Corrected Model	.416(a)	5	.083	5.476	.000
Intercept	180.192	1	180.192	11851.548	.000
alcgroup	.215	4	.054	3.534	.007
cigsgp	.214	1	.214	14.054	.000
Error	6.842	450	.015		
Total	467.881	456			
Corrected Total	7.258	455			

a R Squared = .057 (Adjusted R Squared = .047)

The overall *P* values for alcohol and smoking

Custom Hypothesis Tests Index

1	Contrast Coefficients (L' Matrix)	Simple Contrast (reference category = 1) for alcgroup
	Transformation Coefficients (M Matrix)	Identity Matrix
	Contrast Results (K Matrix)	Zero Matrix
2	Contrast Coefficients (L' Matrix)	Simple Contrast (reference category = 1) for cigsgp
	Transformation Coefficients (M Matrix)	Identity Matrix
	Contrast Results (K Matrix)	Zero Matrix

The reference category is the first category for smokers and drinkers, i.e. light smokers and non–drinkers

Figure 10.6 Output from multiple regression with categorical predictor variables in SPSS

analysis will give a *P* value for the individual comparison of two categories. In Stata, the overall *P* value can be obtained following **regress** by using the **test** command (Fig. 10.5). On the other hand **anova** will not give individual comparisons unless followed by the **regress** command (Fig. 10.7).

In the birthweight example, we have assumed that the effect of birthweight is the same in each category of drinking. The degree by which the effect of smoking varies with alcohol is called an 'interaction'. Interactions can be fitted using analysis of variance procedures and are the default in SPSS with the General Linear Model. We have not fitted an interaction to any of the models in this chapter, and Figure 10.6 shows how to obtain an analysis without fitting the interaction term.

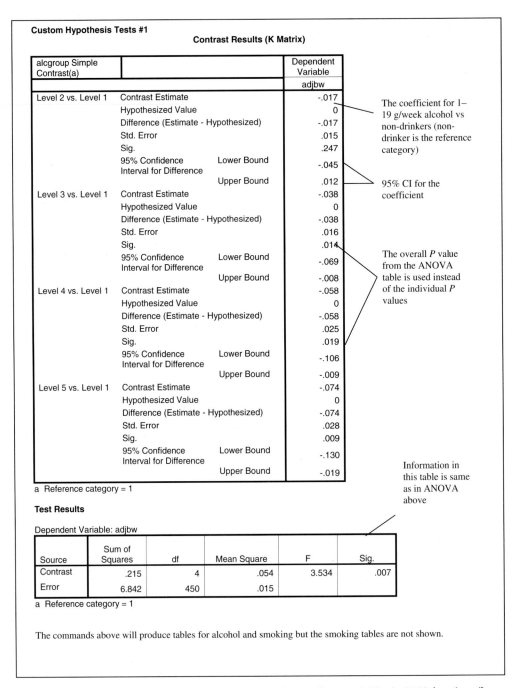

Figure 10.6 Output from multiple regression with categorical predictor variables in SPSS (continued)

10.3.5 **Presenting unadjusted and adjusted estimates**

Sometimes an analysis is performed to investigate several possible predictor variables, and this is followed by a multiple regression analysis to disentangle the effects. In this situation, it may be useful to present both the unadjusted and the adjusted effect estimates to show how much or how little the effect sizes change after other factors are allowed for.

This is the same analysis as in Figure 10.5

cigsgp is the grouping variable for smoking and has two categories, light smokers and heavy smokers. These were coded 1, 2 respectively

alcgroup1 represents five categories of alcohol intake range:, 0, 1–19, 20–49, 50–99, and 100+ g/week. These were coded 5, 4, 3, 2, 1. This is because Stata will take the highest category as the reference and non-drinkers was chosen as the reference.

adjbw is the outcome and represents a standardised birthweight score (birthweight for gestational age)

Further details of these variables are omitted but can be found in Peacock et al. (1991).

```
. anova adjbw cigsgp alcgroup1

              Number of obs =      456      R-squared      =  0.0574
              Root MSE      = .123305      Adj R-squared =  0.0469

     Source |  Partial SS    df       MS           F      Prob > F
------------+----------------------------------------------------
      Model |  .416319047     5  .083263809       5.48     0.0001
            |
     cigsgp |  .213684016     1  .213684016      14.05     0.0002
  alcgroup1 |  .214931901     4  .053732975       3.53     0.0075
            |
   Residual |  6.84185173   450  .015204115
------------+----------------------------------------------------
      Total |  7.25817077   455  .015952024
```

Overall *P* value for smoking is the same as in the table below as there are only two groups.

Overall *P* value for alcohol

```
. regress

     Source |       SS       df       MS              Number of obs =     456
------------+------------------------------         F(  5,    450) =    5.48
      Model |  .416319047     5  .083263809         Prob > F      =  0.0001
   Residual |  6.84185173   450  .015204115         R-squared     =  0.0574
------------+------------------------------         Adj R-squared =  0.0469
      Total |  7.25817077   455  .015952024         Root MSE      =   .1233


      adjbw |     Coef.   Std. Err.      t    P>|t|    [95% Conf. Interval]
------------+---------------------------------------------------------------
      _cons |   1.013439   .0090251   112.29   0.000    .9957021   1.031175
     cigsgp |
          1 |   .0553906   .0147751     3.75   0.000    .0263538   .0844274
          2 |  (dropped)
  alcgroup1 |
          1 |  -.0742407    .028292    -2.62   0.009   -.1298416  -.0186398
          2 |  -.0577793   .0245754    -2.35   0.019   -.1060762  -.0094825
          3 |  -.0382412   .0155193    -2.46   0.014   -.0687405  -.0077419
          4 |  -.0168603   .0145368    -1.16   0.247   -.0454287   .0117081
          5 |  (dropped)
------------+---------------------------------------------------------------
```

Coefficient for 1–19 g/week alcohol vs non-drinkers (non-drinker is the reference category)

Coefficient for light smoking vs heavy smoking (heavy smoking is the reference category)

Continuous variables can be added to the model by using the **cont** option
e.g. . **anova adjbw cigsgp alcgroup1 age, cont(age)**

Figure 10.7 Output from multiple regression with categorical predictor variables using anova in Stata

In Box 10.9 we show how to present such results. These data come from the UKOS study and represent a sub-sample of infants who had a detailed portfolio of lung function assessments at age 12 months. The assessments required complex equipment which was located in one London hospital, and so it was only possible to include infants who were born in or near to London. This particular analysis sought to estimate the effect of gender on lung function since it was suspected that boys have poorer lung function

BOX 10.9 EXAMPLE

Presenting unadjusted and adjusted estimates after a multiple regression analysis

UKOS sub-study of lung function

Aim of study To investigate factors affecting lung function at 12 months in ex-preterm infants.

Study design Cohort study.

Study population Seventy-six preterm infants assessed at age 12 months.

Aim of analysis To estimate the difference in respiratory function between males and females.

Description

Methods section

The difference in lung function between males and females was estimated. Multiple regression was used to adjust the differences between males and females for neonatal factors (birthweight standard deviation score, days ventilated, and oxygen dependency at discharge) and size at assessment (length and weight). Results are presented as unadjusted and adjusted differences with 95% confidence intervals. Percentage difference was also calculated to facilitate comparison of sex effects among the different lung function measures.

Results section

Table. Mean lung function in males ($N=42$) and females ($N=34$) before and after adjustment for predictive neonatal factors

Outcome	Male Mean (SD)	Female Mean (SD)	Difference (95%CI) male–female	Adjusted difference[1] (95%CI) male–female	% reduction[2]
FRC pleth (ml/kg)	244.2 (50.8)	213.6 (34.5)	30.6 (9.8, 51.5)	37.8 (13.7, 61.9)	17.7%
Raw (kPa/[l/s])	3.79 (1.58)	2.81 (1.01)	0.98 (0.31, 1.64)	0.36 (−0.40, 1.12)	12.8%
SGaw (1/[kPa.s])	1.28 (0.45)	1.93 (0.61)	−0.65 (−0.90, −0.40)	−0.51 (−0.80, −0.21)	26.4%
FRCHe (ml)	212.4 (45.6)	201.3 (35.0)	11.1 (−8.3, 30.6)	19.9 (−1.8, 41.6)	9.9%

[1]difference between males and females adjusted for birthweight standard deviation score, days ventilated, oxygen dependency at discharge, length, and weight at time of measurement

[2]Calculated as $100 \times$ (adjusted difference)/female mean

Mean lung function was lower for males than females for all four measures, and all except FRCHe were statistically significant. After adjusting for birth factors and current size, the differences were similar although FRCHe and Raw were not significant. The size of difference in lung function measures between males and females varied between 10% and 26% (table).

Discussion points

The reduction in lung function for boys is substantial and is not fully explained by differences in neonatal characteristics or current size. The non-significance for FRCHe and Raw is likely to be due to small sample size as the estimated reductions were still quite large, lying between 10% and 13%.

than girls, but this had not been characterised in a very young ex-preterm group.

Stata and SPSS outputs have not been shown since these are similar to those shown earlier. By presenting the unadjusted and adjusted estimates side by side, the effect of adjusting can be seen. For some measures the difference between males and females increases after adjustment, while for others it decreases. Where estimates remain of similar size after adjustment, it indicates that the effect is not due to confounding by the factors allowed for. Conversely, if an estimate decreases after adjustment, then this suggests that the original effect observed was at least partly due to other factors.

Also note that in this example there are several outcomes which are measured on different scales. To facilitate comparison between these, we have presented the male–female difference as a percentage of the female mean value. This allows the reader to compare the effect of sex on the different measures, even though each is measured on a different scale.

10.4 **Logistic regression**

10.4.1 **Introduction**

In the previous section we used multiple regression to examine the relationship between a continuous outcome and several predictor variables. Logistic regression can be used to carry out similar analyses for binary outcome variables. Box 10.10 summarises the main features and assumptions of the method.

BOX 10.10 INFORMATION

Logistic regression

Null hypothesis There is no relationship between the outcome and the predictor variable

Note This hypothesis applies separately to each predictor variable in the model

Use for
- Binary outcome and several predictor variables
- Predictors can be continuous, binary, or categorical

Assumptions
- For continuous predictors only, the relationship is linear on the logit scale.
- Large sample method. Rule of thumb is that the analysis requires at least 10 positives and 10 negatives per predictor variable (Peduzzi *et al.* 1996)

Deviations from assumptions
- If the relationship is not linear then either a transformation of the predictor variable may be used to model the actual relationship or the predictor variable may be categorised into several groups
- If the sample is too small, use an exact method (not available in Stata or standard SPSS) or reduce number of predictors

---

BOX 10.11 HELPFUL TIPS

Logistic regression: interpretation of coefficients

Log odds ratios

- Coefficients from logistic regression are log odds ratios
- These must be back-transformed (take exponential) to give odds ratios
- Stata and SPSS will do this for you, or use calculator
- Below we assume that coefficients have been back-transformed

Binary predictor variables

- Odds ratio for outcome in the two levels of predictor variable. For example, if the outcome is death and the predictor variable is smoking, then we obtain the ratio of odds of dying in smokers vs non-smokers
- Note that it is important to know the coding for the variable under consideration to be able to determine which direction the difference is in
- If all variables are coded 0=no,1=yes, then in Stata and SPSS the odds ratio will be the odds of the outcome in the 'yes' group divided by the odds of the outcome in the 'no' group (yes/no)

Categorical predictor variables

- Odds ratio for outcome in given category divided by odds of outcome in reference category
- Stata uses the category with the lowest code as the reference category, while SPSS allows the user to choose the lowest or highest code

Continuous predictor variables

- Odds ratio is the change in odds of outcome for a unit change in predictor
- For example, if the outcome was death and the predictor was the number of packs of cigarettes smoked per day, then the odds ratio would be for 2 packs/day vs 1 pack/day. This is the same as 3 packs/day vs 2 packs/day etc.
- If the odds ratio was 1.5, then 4 packs/day vs 1 pack/day would be obtained by taking $1.5 \times 1.5 \times 1.5 = 1.5^3 = 3.4$

The strength of the relationship is estimated by the odds ratio which will be adjusted for other variables fitted in the model. When there is only one predictor variable the odds ratio produced from the logistic regression, will be the same as that calculated directly from the 2×2 table (Box 7.9). For binary predictor variables it is important to be clear about the direction of the effect (Box 10.11). For continuous predictors the odds ratio obtained is the odds of outcome for a unit change in predictor. More details are given in Box 10.11.

To illustrate the presentation of logistic regression, we will use data from the UKOS study. The data come from a paediatrician follow-up at 12 months, and this analysis looks at the relationship between neonatal factors and whether or not chest medicines were prescribed at 12 months. Eight neonatal variables were examined in unifactorial analyses initially to see if they were associated with prescribed chest medicines. The four variables that were significant at the 5% level (sex, multiple birth, oxygen dependency at 36 weeks post-menstrual age, oxygen dependency at hospital discharge) were then put in a logistic regression model to try to disentangle the effects. Figures 10.8 and 10.9 show the Stata and SPSS outputs.

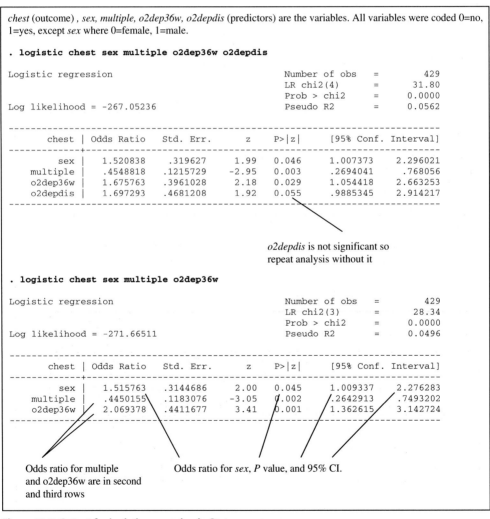

chest (outcome), *sex, multiple, o2dep36w, o2depdis* (predictors) are the variables. All variables were coded 0=no, 1=yes, except *sex* where 0=female, 1=male.

```
. logistic chest sex multiple o2dep36w o2depdis

Logistic regression                             Number of obs   =       429
                                                LR chi2(4)      =     31.80
                                                Prob > chi2     =    0.0000
Log likelihood = -267.05236                     Pseudo R2       =    0.0562

-------------------------------------------------------------------------
   chest |  Odds Ratio   Std. Err.      z    P>|z|    [95% Conf. Interval]
---------+---------------------------------------------------------------
     sex |   1.520838    .319627     1.99   0.046    1.007373    2.296021
multiple |   .4548818    .1215729   -2.95   0.003    .2694041     .768056
o2dep36w |   1.675763    .3961028    2.18   0.029    1.054418    2.663253
o2depdis |   1.697293    .4681208    1.92   0.055    .9885345    2.914217
-------------------------------------------------------------------------
```

o2depdis is not significant so repeat analysis without it

```
. logistic chest sex multiple o2dep36w

Logistic regression                             Number of obs   =       429
                                                LR chi2(3)      =     28.34
                                                Prob > chi2     =    0.0000
Log likelihood = -271.66511                     Pseudo R2       =    0.0496

-------------------------------------------------------------------------
   chest |  Odds Ratio   Std. Err.      z    P>|z|    [95% Conf. Interval]
---------+---------------------------------------------------------------
     sex |   1.515763    .3144686    2.00   0.045    1.009337    2.276283
multiple |   .4450155    .1183076   -3.05   0.002    .2642913    .7493202
o2dep36w |   2.069378    .4411677    3.41   0.001    1.362615    3.142724
-------------------------------------------------------------------------
```

Odds ratio for multiple and o2dep36w are in second and third rows

Odds ratio for *sex*, *P* value, and 95% CI.

Figure 10.8 Output for logistic regression in Stata

chest (outcome) , *sex, multiple, o2dep36w, o2depdis* (predictors) are the variables. All variables were coded 0=no, 1=yes, except *sex* where 0=female, 1=male.
Select 'Analyze'
Select 'Regression'
Select 'Binary Logistic'
Move *chest* into the 'Dependent' and *sex, multiple, o2dep36w and o2depdis* into the 'Covariates' boxes
Select 'Options' and tick the 'CI for Exp(B)' box

Only the relevant output has been shown here

Block 1: Model=Enter

Omnibus Tests of Model Coefficients

		Chi-square	df	Sig.
Step 1	Step	31.796	4	.000
	Block	31.796	4	.000
	Model	31.796	4	.000

Model Summary

Step	-2 Log likelihood	Cox & Snell R Square	Nagelkerke R Square
1	534.105(a)	.072	.098

a Estimation terminated at iteration number 4 because parameter estimates changed by less than .001.

Variables in the Equation

		B	S.E.	Wald	df	Sig.	Exp(B)	95.0% C.I.for EXP(B)	
								Lower	Upper
Step 1(a)	sex	.419	.210	3.980	1	.046	1.521	1.007	2.296
	multiple	-.788	.267	8.687	1	.003	.455	.269	.768
	o2dep36w	.516	.236	4.770	1	.029	1.676	1.054	2.663
	o2depdis	.529	.276	3.679	1	.055	1.697	.989	2.914
	Constant	-.956	.198	23.240	1	.000	.385		

a Variable(s) entered on step 1: sex, multiple, o2dep36w, o2depdis.

o2depdis is not significant so repeat analysis without it

Only last table of the output shown for the analysis without *02depdis*

Variables in the Equation

		B	S.E.	Wald	df	Sig.	Exp(B)	95.0% C.I.for EXP(B)	
								Lower	Upper
Step 1(a)	sex	.416	.207	4.019	1	.045	1.516	1.009	2.276
	multiple	-.810	.266	9.275	1	.002	.445	.264	.749
	o2dep36w	.727	.213	11.637	1	.001	2.069	1.363	3.143
	Constant	-.958	.197	23.673	1	.000	.383		

a Variable(s) entered on step 1: sex, multiple, o2dep36w.

P values and odds ratio for *multiple* and *o2dep36w* are in second and third rows

P value for *sex*, odds ratio and 95% CI

Figure 10.9 Output for logistic regression in SPSS

10.4.2 **Presenting the results of logistic regression**

Box 10.12 shows how to present the results. We have given the number and percentage of babies in the whole group who were prescribed chest medicines. This gives an estimate of the overall risk and shows that the number of events is sufficiently large for a robust logistic regression analysis. We have not presented summary statistics for the study because of lack of space but are assuming that these would be presented before the logistic regression. We have

given the odds ratio, 95% confidence interval, and *P* value in a table.

We have indicated the direction of effect for sex (male/female). For the yes/no variables, we have assumed that the odds ratio is for yes vs no. In the description we have indicated the size of effect and stated that the odds ratios are adjusted for the other variables in the model to distinguish these results from ordinary variable-by-variable results (unadjusted results). We will give an example of presenting unadjusted and adjusted results together later in this chapter. (Section 10.4.4)

BOX 10.12 EXAMPLE

Presenting the results for logistic regression

UKOS study

Aim of study To assess respiratory health at 12 months following very premature birth.

Study design Follow-up of surviving babies from a randomised controlled trial.

Study population 429 surviving infants.

Aim of analysis To investigate the effect of neonatal factors on use of chest medicines at 12 months.

Description

Methods section

The combined effect of four neonatal variables which were significantly related to the use of chest medicines at 12 months (sex, single or multiple birth, oxygen dependency at 36 weeks PMA, oxygen dependency at discharge) were investigated using logistic regression. Results are presented as odds ratios and 95% confidence intervals.

Results section

Table. Adjusted[1] odds ratios for effects of neonatal variables on use of chest medicines at 12 months in 429 infants

Variable	Odds ratio	95% CI	P value
Sex (male/female)	1.52	1.01, 2.28	0.045
Multiple birth	0.45	0.26, 0.75	0.002
O$_2$ dependency at 36 weeks PMA[2]	2.07	1.36, 3.14	0.001

[1] Each odds ratio is adjusted for all other variables in the table

[2] PMA, post-menstrual age

165 babies (38%) were prescribed chest medicines at 12 months of age. The proportion prescribed chest medicine was higher in males than females (45% vs 32%), lower in multiple births than singletons (25% vs 42%), and higher in those who were oxygen dependent at 36 weeks PMA (46% vs 28%) and in those who were oxygen dependent at discharge (55% vs 34%).

When the four significant neonatal variables were analysed together, oxygen dependency at discharge became non-significant (OR 1.70, 95% CI 0.99, 2.91) but the other three remained significant. After adjustment, male sex was associated with a 50% increase in odds of use of chest medicines, while multiple birth was associated with a halving of the odds. Oxygen dependency at 36 weeks was associated with over a twofold increase in odds of prescription of chest medicines.

BOX 10.13 INFORMATION

Categorical variables in logistic regression using Stata and SPSS

Stata

◆ Use **xi:logistic** (as in Figure 10.10) to identify the categorical variables

◆ Uses the lowest category as the reference

◆ Need to use **test** command to obtain overall *P* value (Figure 10.10)

SPSS

◆ Must use **categorical** option to identify categorical variables

◆ Can choose reference category to be first or last

◆ Gives overall *P* value by default

Both programs

◆ Binary variables need not be identified as categorical

◆ The reference category should not contain a small number of observations

◆ The reference category should be one that makes sense; for example, it is more reasonable to choose non-drinkers than heavy drinkers as a reference category

10.4.3 Presenting logistic regression with categorical predictor variables

The main features of presenting categorical variables in logistic regression are similar to those for multiple regression (section 10.3.3). Overall *P* values should be presented and care needs to be taken to obtain and describe the appropriate reference category (Box 10.13). Both SPSS and Stata assume that predictor variables are continuous unless otherwise specified as in Figures 10.10 and 10.11.

To illustrate, we will investigate the relationship between nausea and smoking and social class from the birthweight study. This is related to the analysis shown in section 8.5. In the unifactorial analysis we used relative risk to describe the relationships. Here we will use odds ratios because the analysis is more straightforward than one which attempts to adjust the relative risks, especially as the outcome is common (see Box 7.9). Smoking habit is divided into three categories: non smokers, light smokers, and heavy smokers. The Stata and SPSS outputs are shown in Figures 10.10 and 10.11 and the presentation is show in Box 10.14.

We have presented the odds ratios, 95% confidence intervals, and *P* values. The overall *P* value for smoking is given alongside the reference category and the 95% confidence intervals are given for each comparison. The direction of the effects is obvious because we have indicated the reference category against which all other categories are compared. Note that in this example we have explicitly indicated the reference category by putting an odds ratio of 1.0 next to it. If space was limited, we could have simply used a footnote to show which the reference categories were, as we did in Box 10.8.

We have described the direction of the effects and stated that these are adjusted effects. It would be important to say this if there were any possibility of ambiguity, for example when unadjusted and adjusted effects are described together. If it is obvious that the odds ratios are adjusted, then a simple statement that all effect estimates are adjusted for all other variables in the model is sufficient.

We have described the results in terms which do not imply causality since this is an observational study where the outcome and exposures are occurring concurrently. It would, of course, be wrong to state, or imply, that this analysis shows that smoking and manual social class protect against nausea in pregnancy. The relationship *may* be causal, but it is more likely that smoking and manual social class are markers for women who tend not to get nausea for other reasons. Another possibility is that that women who have nausea stop smoking. This study and this analysis cannot distinguish between these possibilities, and we have to be careful how we describe and present the results so as not to mislead the reader.

The variables used in this analysis are *nausea1 smoker1* and *socialclass. nausea1* is coded 0,1 (no/yes) and *smoker1* is coded 0,1,2 (non-smoker, light smoker, heavy smoker). *socialclass* is coded 0,1 (non-manual/manual)
Select 'Analyze'
Select 'Regression'
Select 'Binary Logistic'
Move *nausea1* into the 'Dependent' and *smoker1* and *socialclass* into the 'Covariates' boxes
Select 'Options' and tick the 'CI for Exp(B)' box
Select 'Categorical'
For each variable highlight the variable and then select 'Simple' from the contrast list and 'first' as the reference category. Click 'Change'

Only the relevant output has been shown here

Case Processing Summary

Unweighted Cases(a)		N	Percent
Selected Cases	Included in Analysis	1469	97.1
	Missing Cases	44	2.9
	Total	1513	100.0
Unselected Cases		0	.0
Total		1513	100.0

a If weight is in effect, see classification table for the total number of cases.

Block 1: Method=Enter

Omnibus Tests of Model Coefficients

		Chi-square	df	Sig.
Step 1	Step	24.890	3	.000
	Block	24.890	3	.000
	Model	24.890	3	.000

Odds ratio for light smokers vs non-smokers (reference category)

Model Summary

Step	-2 Log likelihood	Cox & Snell R Square	Nagelkerke R Square
1	1467.744(a)	.017	.026

a Estimation terminated at iteration number 4 because parameter estimates changed by less than .001.

Variables in the Equation

		B	S.E.	Wald	df	Sig.	Exp(B)	95.0% C.I.for EXP(B)	
								Lower	Upper
Step 1(a)	smoker1			17.399	2	.000			
	smoker1(1)	-.523	.153	11.764	1	.001	.593	.439	.799
	smoker1(2)	-.633	.200	9.991	1	.002	.531	.359	.786
	socialclass(1)	-.319	.158	4.076	1	.043	.727	.534	.991
	Constant	1.077	.085	159.507	1	.000	2.934		

a Variable(s) entered on step 1: smoker1, socialclass.

P value for overall effect of smoking

P value for social class and odds ratio (95% CI) for manual vs non-manual (reference category)

Figure 10.11 Output for logistic regression with categorical predictor variables in SPSS

BOX 10.14 EXAMPLE

Presenting logistic regression with categorical predictor variables

Birthweight study

Aim of study To investigate symptoms and health problems in pregnancy.

Study design Cohort study.

Study population 1469 pregnant women booking in one hospital.

Aim of analysis To investigate the relationship between nausea in pregnancy and mother's smoking and social class.

Description

Methods section

The effects of smoking and social class on nausea in early pregnancy were investigated using logistic regression. Results are presented as odds ratios and 95% confidence intervals.

Results section

Table. Adjusted odds ratios for the effects of smoking and social class on nausea in early pregnancy in 1469 women

Variable	Odds ratio[1]	95% CI	P value
Smoking			
Non-smoker[2]	1.0		<0.001
Light smoker	0.59	0.44, 0.80	
Heavy smoker	0.53	0.36, 0.79	
Social class			
Non-manual[2]	1.0		0.04
Manual	0.73	0.53, 0.99	

[1] Adjusted for the other variables in the table

[2] reference category

Overall, the majority of women (1167/1469, 79%) reported nausea during the first trimester of pregnancy. However, nausea was significantly less common in smokers than in non-smokers (72% vs 83%) and was less common in women in manual than in non-manual occupation (73% vs 81%).

   After mutual adjustment, both smoking and social class remained significantly associated with nausea in pregnancy. After adjustment for social class, both light and heavy smoking were associated with reduced odds of nausea compared with not smoking. After adjustment for smoking, women in manual occupations had reduced odds of nausea than those in non-manual occupations (table).

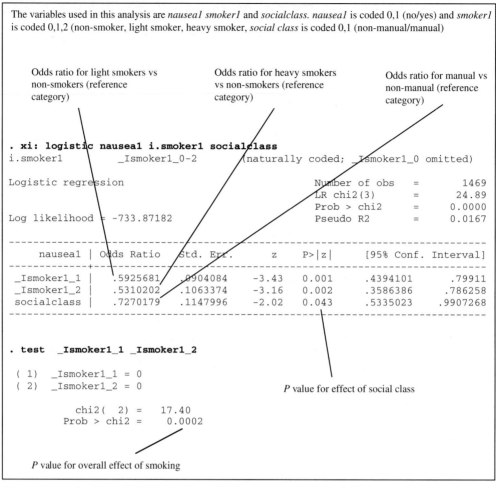

Figure 10.10 Output for logistic regression with categorical predictor variables

10.4.4 Presenting unadjusted and adjusted odds ratios

Sometimes it can be informative to present the unadjusted estimates as well as adjusted estimates obtained from a multifactorial analysis. This can be useful to show how estimates change after adjustment. Box 10.15 shows an extract of a table from the UKOS study which was reporting on the predictors of respiratory symptoms in infants. Several variables were associated with adverse symptoms when examined in unifactorial analyses, and it was interesting to see that the strengths of the relationships did not change much after mutual adjustment. As commented in the box, this suggests that

the predictors were acting independently of each other. If alternatively, for example, one estimate had been much smaller after adjustment, this would have suggested that part of its observed effect when examined alone was in fact due to the other variables in the model.

When reporting unadjusted and adjusted estimates together, it may not be necessary to give confidence intervals for the unadjusted estimates if space is limited, but confidence intervals should be given for the adjusted estimates. Another example of presenting unadjusted and adjusted estimates was given in Box 5.5.

BOX 10.15 EXAMPLE

Presenting unadjusted and adjusted logistic regression

Description

Results section

Table. Factors related to cough and wheeze reported at both 6 and 12 months of age estimated in logistic regression analysis

Outcome	Predictor variables	Unadjusted OR	Adjusted OR	Adjusted (95%CI)
Cough	Sex: boy	1.80	1.83	1.11, 3.02
	Oxygen dependent at discharge	2.01	1.76	1.00, 3.11
	Live in rented accommodation	1.96	1.67	1.02, 2.73
	Older siblings aged < 5 years	1.70	2.25	1.34, 3.80
Wheeze	Multiple birth	0.36	0.37	0.18, 0.77
	Oxygen dependent at 36 weeks PMA	2.43	2.74	1.55, 4.83
	Pet ownership	0.42	0.43	0.21, 0.87
	Older siblings aged < 5 years	1.54	1.98	1.13, 3.49

Four factors were significantly associated with cough. Male sex, oxygen dependency at hospital discharge, living in rented accommodation, and having older siblings under the age of 5 years were associated with 1.7- to 2-fold increases in odds of cough. For wheeze, predictive factors were oxygen dependency at 36 weeks and older siblings, showing 1.5-to over 2-fold increases in odds. Multiple birth and pet ownership showed inverse (protective) associations with wheeze. Unadjusted and adjusted odds ratios were very similar.

Discussion points

The similarity of the unadjusted and adjusted odds ratios suggests that these factors are acting independently of each other.

(Greenough *et al.* 2005)

10.5 Further reading

The references given in Box 10.16 are those that we have found particularly useful for the specific topics listed.

BOX 10.16 INFORMATION

Further information on statistical methods

One-way analysis of variance

Altman (1991, Chapter 9), Armitage *et al.* (2002, Chapter 8), Bland (2000, Chapter 10), Kirkwood and Sterne (2003, Chapter 9)

Multiple comparisons

Altman (1991, Chapter 9), Armitage *et al.* (2002, Chapter 8), Bland (2000, Chapter 9)

Multiple regression

Altman (1991, Chapter 12), Armitage *et al.* (2002, Chapter 11), Bland (2000, Chapter 17), Kirkwood and Sterne (2003, Chapter 11)

Logistic regression

Altman (1991, Chapter 12), Armitage *et al.* (2002, Chapter 14), Bland (2000, Chapter 17), Kirkwood and Sterne (2003, Ch 19, 20)

Chapter summary

Multifactorial analyses

- Plan the analysis beforehand and present what you find even if results are not significant
- Present summary statistics for the variables included which are appropriate to the analysis
- Make sure categorical and continuous variables are specified correctly in the statistical program used
- Make and report on appropriate adjustment for any multiple comparisons
- Present adjusted slopes, adjusted difference in means, or adjusted odds ratios as appropriate, with their 95% CIs
- Report all the variables included in the models fitted
- Unless it is obvious, specify how the variables have been modelled. For example, age could be modelled as a continuous variable with a linear relationship, as a quadratic relationship, or treated as categorical etc.
- Clearly state reference categories and direction of differences
- Give the overall *P* value for a categorical variable with more than two groups
- Report any transformations of the data
- Check that the assumptions of the method hold, although this is not usually reported in papers and reports

CHAPTER 11

Survival analysis

11.1 Introduction

In the peripheral vascular disease study (Box 7.2), we have simply classified subjects into those who died and those who survived. Another way of looking at the data is to see how long patients survived. Although commonly referred to as 'survival' analysis, these methods are more generally described as 'time-to-event' analysis. They take into account the different lengths of time subjects have been followed up without experiencing an event (see Box 11.1).

In studies where all subjects have experienced an event and no subjects are lost to follow-up, the time to event can be analysed using methods described earlier in the book (Chapter 7). Since time to event is often highly skewed, a transformation followed by a *t* test or a rank test such as the Mann–Whitney *U* test may be appropriate. For example, in a trial of a drug to resolve symptoms for sore throat in healthy individuals, all participants would experience resolution of symptoms (the event), and so the length of time to resolution could be directly compared.

In this chapter we will describe the Kaplan–Meier methods for displaying the survival curve and estimating survival rates, the log rank test, and Cox regression. There are several other methods of estimating survival rates but most give similar results. For a more detailed discussion of various

Uses of survival methods

Used for time to any event
For example, time to recovery, time to conception, time to recurrence of disease, time to death, time to first cardiovascular event (fatal or non-fatal).

Number of events per person
Standard statistical procedures assume that one event per person is included so if a person could have more than one event (e.g. non-fatal cardiovascular event), then the time to a specific event (e.g. the first event) can be analysed.

Multiple events per person can be analysed, but this is not straightforward and details are omitted here. We recommend seeking statistical help if you want to analyse multiple events.

Censored observations
Survival methods make allowance for incomplete follow-up of subjects. All subjects who have not experienced the event are 'censored' at the last time their status was known (e.g. the last time they were known to be alive). They contribute to the number of patients 'at risk' of the event up until this point.

Reasons for censoring might include
(1) died from unrelated cause

(2) died from unrelated accident

(3) the event did not occur before the end of study period

(4) moved away

(5) withdrew from study

Assumptions
'Censored' individuals are assumed to have the same probability of the event in the period after they left the study as those still remaining.

This is likely to be true for reasons 1–3 above but may not be with reasons 4 and 5. It is possible that subjects who moved away may be fitter and so have a lower probability of the event. Subjects who withdraw from a study might do so because of treatment failure or success, and so again might be different from those who remain.

Using life tables in Stata and SPSS

Life tables
The life table method assumes that the event is known to occur within a time period rather than taking place at a specific time.

This method in Stata and SPSS gives the same survival rates as Kaplan–Meier methods when survival times are not grouped. In SPSS the user needs to set 'display time interval' to be the smallest time unit used (e.g. 1 month if survival is measured in months).

Events taking place within first time period
In Stata, **ltable** may be useful where events are recorded as taking place at the same time as recruitment. For example, in the early pregnancy study, time of miscarriage was reported in whole weeks. Therefore it was possible for a woman to be recruited in the same week as she miscarried. In Stata, Kaplan–Meier methods would exclude these women while the **ltable** command includes them.

Graphs without marking censored observations
In SPSS, the KaplanMeier survival curves display censored observations as in Figure 11.2. The **Life Tables** command with a small 'display time interval' will display the same curves without marking the censored observations.

Missing values in SPSS
In SPSS, subjects with missing time values are not excluded by default. Use 'Select cases' to exclude these subjects prior to analysis.

methods see Campbell (2001) and Parmar and Machin (1995).

An alternative to the Kaplan–Meier method is the life table method, which assumes that events are known to take place within a time period rather than taking place at a certain time. If life table methods are used with a small interval, they will give the same results as Kaplan–Meier methods. There are a few situations where the life table procedures in Stata or SPSS may be useful and these are given in Box 11.2.

11.1.1 Description of the study sample

The report of the results of survival analysis should start with a description of the sample. This should include the total sample size, the total number of events, and the average (mean or median) follow-up time, as well as some measure of variability in the follow-up times, such as the range. For a randomised trial, these should be reported for each group separately. The report should state the reasons why subjects are lost to follow-up or censored, showing if possible that the reasons are unrelated to the probability of an event occurring (see Box 11.1). In the peripheral vascular disease study most of the censored subjects had been recruited later in the study and so had a shorter time in the study. In a trial, patients may drop out if the treatment is not effective. These patients should be regarded as 'failures' and not as 'censored' observations.

11.1.2 Kaplan–Meier survival curves

Kaplan–Meier survival curves are a useful way of summarising the survival, or time-to-event characteristics, of one or more groups of individuals and should be presented wherever possible. Box 11.3 gives useful tips on drawing these curves in Stata and SPSS.

Survival curves for peripheral vascular disease in patients with and without diabetes were produced using the Kaplan–Meier method (Box 11.4). Figures 11.1 and 11.2 show how to draw similar curves with Stata and SPSS. The graphs show that subjects with diabetes tended to die sooner than those without diabetes.

Survival curves are always shown as a series of steps, with the horizontal lines between steps indicating that the probability of survival remains constant between events.

When describing or interpreting a Kaplan–Meier curve, care should be taken not place too much emphasis on the right-hand side of the graph if the numbers at risk are small, or only a small proportion of the original sample remain in the study. The graph in Box 11.4 has been curtailed when the numbers of subjects at risk fell below 5 (Box 11.3). Where the number of subjects is large and they have been followed up for differing lengths of time, it is recommended that the graph

is curtailed when only 10% of the original sample is still at risk.

The numbers at risk are displayed at regular time points. This was done by editing the graph after it was produced in Stata. It shows that the number at risk is much smaller in the diabetes, group, especially on the right-hand side of the graph.

An alternative to displaying the numbers at risk is to show where observations have been censored. The graph in Figure 11.2 shows tick marks at each censored observation. It indicates that most censoring took place late on in the study, probably because the subjects were still alive when the study ended.

months is the follow-up time inmonths
outcome is coded 0 = alive, 1 = dead; any value greater than 0 will be interpreted as 'failure' i.e. death
diabetes is coded 1 = diabetic, 0 = non-diabetic

stset describes the survival variables in the data. This command needs to executed only once and is then followed by any of the analysis commands in this figure, or in Figures 11.4 or 11.6. Note that if the data are changed in any way, this command will need to be re-run.

```
.stset months, failure(outcome)
```

11 subjects had missing follow-up times. Any subjects with follow-up time equal to entry time (here 0) will also be excluded (see Box11.2)

```
     failure event:  outcome != 0 & outcome < .
obs. time interval:  (0, months]
 exit on or before:  failure
```

```
-------------------------------------------------------------------
      121   total obs.
       11   event time missing (months>=.)           PROBABLE ERROR
-------------------------------------------------------------------
      110   obs. remaining, representing
       61   failures in single record/single failure data
     5622   total analysis time at risk, at risk from t =        0
                           earliest observed entry t =        0
                              last observed exit t =     104.5
```

61 patients died out of a total of 110

```
. sts graph,by(diabetes) ytitle(Probability of survival) xtitle(Time in months)
```

```
        failure _d:  outcome
  analysis time _t:  months
```

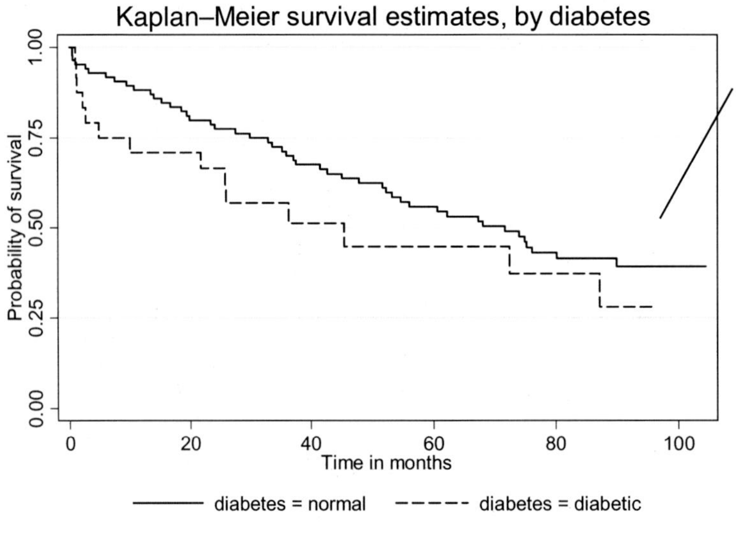

Among diabetics, no patients were followed up for more than 96 months. The graph in Box 11.4 has been curtailed at 84 months where numbersat risk fell to below 5

Figure 11.1 Kaplan–Meier curve in Stata

months is the follow-up time in months
outcome is coded 0 = alive,1 = dead
diabetes is coded 1 = diabetic,0 = non-diabetic
Select 'Analyze'
Select 'Survival'
Select 'Kaplan–Meier'
Move *months* to 'Time' box; *outcome* to 'Status' box; Select 'Define Event', next to 'Single value' put 1
Move *diabetes* to 'Factor' box
Select 'Options' and tick 'Survival' under 'Plots'

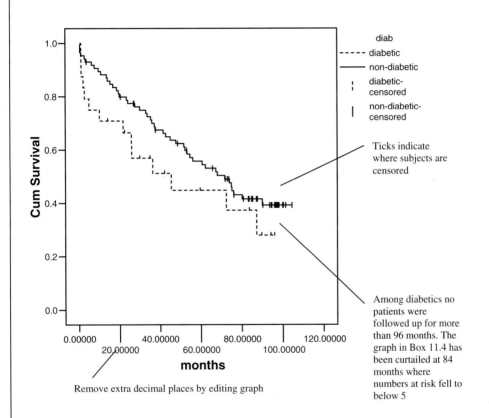

To curtail the graph early at 84 recode all cases with follow-up greater than 84 months as censored at 84 months.

Figure 11.2 Kaplan–Meier curve in SPSS

BOX 11.4 EXAMPLE

Presenting Kaplan–Meier analysis

Peripheral vascular disease study

Aim of study To assess the long-term survival of patients with peripheral vascular disease (PVD) and to investigate the impact of the presence of risk factors on mortality.

Study design Cohort study.

Patient population Consecutive patients with PVD and intermittent claudication who were referred for angiography, and found to have angiographic evidence of PVD.

Aim of analysis To compare survival rates in those with and without risk factors, including diabetes.

Description

Methods section

Survival rates are expressed as the percentage surviving for 5 years calculated using the Kaplan–Meier method. Kaplan–Meier curves comparing diabetics and non-diabetics are shown up to 7 years follow-up. The log rank test was used to test the difference between survival curves. All analyses were carried out in Stata version 8.

Results section

A total of 110 subjects were included in this analysis. Mean follow-up time of survivors was 6.1 years; range 14 days to 8.7 years. Thirty-five men and 26 women (55%) died. The Kaplan–Meier curve shows that patients with diabetes have lower survival rates (figure). The 5-year survival rate was 45%, 95% CI (23% to 65%) among those with diabetes and 56% (44% to 66%) among non-diabetics. The log rank test gave $P = 0.19$.

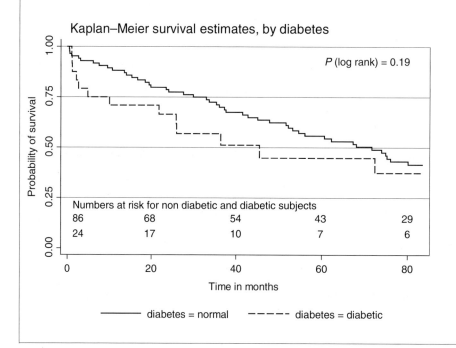

Kaplan–Meier survival estimates, by diabetes

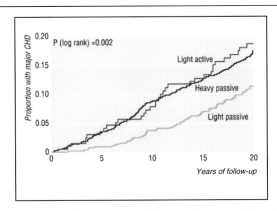

Proportion of men with major CHD by years of follow-up in each smoking group.

'Light passive' refers to lowest quarter of cotinine concentration among non-smokers (0–0.7 ng/ml), 'heavy passive' to upper three-quarters of cotinine concentration combined (0.8 – 14.0 ng/ml), 'light active' to men smoking 1–9 cigarettes a day.

(Whincup *et al. BMJ*, 2004; **329**: 200. Reproduced with permission from the BMJ Publishing Group.)

Figure 11.3 Kaplan–Meier curve plotted upwards to show differences between groups that have low event rates

Box 11.4 also displays the result of the log rank test (described in detail in section 11.3). The log rank test has been included as an indication of the statistical uncertainty in comparing survival in the two groups. Alternative approaches would be to include the estimated hazard ratio with its 95% CI (section 11.4), or to show error bars at regular points on the curve. The error bars could relate to either the standard error of the estimate of survival or the confidence interval, but the authors should make clear which has been used. For a fuller discussion see Pocock *et al.* (2002).

Although we have only analysed two groups here, the Kaplan–Meier method can be used for three or more groups as in Figure 11.3.

11.1.3 Low event rates

If the event rates are less than 30%, the curves will be confined to the top third of the graph and important differences in event rates may not be visible. Figure 11.3 shows a Kaplan–Meier curve for the proportion of subjects suffering from a major coronary heart disease event, according to their exposure to passive smoking, and compared with a group of light smokers. At the 20 year follow-up,

less than 20% of light active smokers had experienced an event, and the rates were even lower for the other groups. If the graph had been plotted downwards, as in Box 11.4, the curves would have been confined to the top fifth of the graph and differences between the groups would be difficult to see. Therefore the graph has been plotted upwards, with the end of the scale at 0.20, just above the 20-year value for the group with the highest mortality. The alternative is to plot downwards with a break in the axes, but it is preferable to use an upwards plot if this is possible. For further discussion of presenting survival plots in clinical trials see Pocock *et al.* (2002).

11.2 Kaplan–Meier estimates of survival rates

The survival rate at a chosen time should be presented for each group with the 95% confidence interval as in Box 11.4. It is useful to decide in advance which time point(s) to present. This may be consistent with convention; for example, most cancer studies report 5-year survival rates. The proportions should be calculated after taking censored observations into account, such as those produced

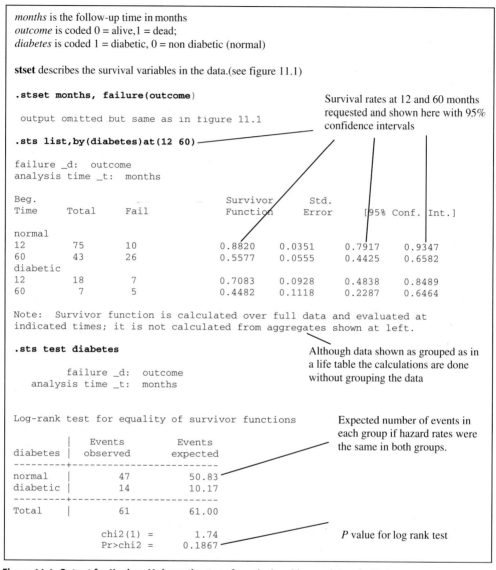

months is the follow-up time in months
outcome is coded 0 = alive,1 = dead;
diabetes is coded 1 = diabetic, 0 = non diabetic (normal)

stset describes the survival variables in the data.(see figure 11.1)

```
.stset months, failure(outcome)

   output omitted but same as in figure 11.1

.sts list,by(diabetes)at(12 60)

failure _d:  outcome
analysis time _t:   months

Beg.                                 Survivor      Std.
Time        Total      Fail          Function      Error        [95% Conf. Int.]

normal
12          75         10            0.8820        0.0351       0.7917       0.9347
60          43         26            0.5577        0.0555       0.4425       0.6582
diabetic
12          18         7             0.7083        0.0928       0.4838       0.8489
60          7          5             0.4482        0.1118       0.2287       0.6464

Note:   Survivor function is calculated over full data and evaluated at
indicated times; it is not calculated from aggregates shown at left.

.sts test diabetes

         failure _d:  outcome
    analysis time _t:  months


Log-rank test for equality of survivor functions

           |  Events           Events
diabetes   |  observed         expected
-----------+---------------------------
normal     |     47             50.83
diabetic   |     14             10.17
-----------+---------------------------
Total      |     61             61.00

           chi2(1) =        1.74
           Pr>chi2 =      0.1867
```

Survival rates at 12 and 60 months requested and shown here with 95% confidence intervals

Although data shown as grouped as in a life table the calculations are done without grouping the data

Expected number of events in each group if hazard rates were the same in both groups.

P value for log rank test

Figure 11.4 Output for Kaplan–Meier estimates of survival and log rank test in Stata

by the Kaplan–Meier method. Care should be taken when comparing survival rates and only a few points should be compared.

Figures 11.4 and 11.5 show the outputs from Stata and SPSS. SPSS does not produce the 95% confidence interval directly but only the standard errors, from which the approximate confidence interval can be calculated as shown in Figure 11.5. This method relies on a large-sample Normal approximation and works reasonably well if the probabilities are between 0.2 and 0.8. If values outside the range 0 to 1 are obtained, this is an indication that there are insufficient data for the assumptions to hold. Stata uses a more exact method which is more difficult to calculate by hand. Box 11.4 uses the figures produced by Stata. Proportions have been multiplied by 100 to give percentages in the presentation.

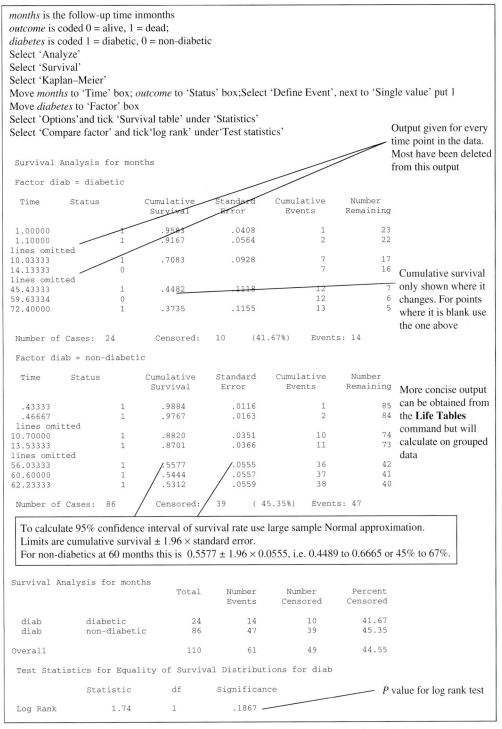

months is the follow-up time in months
outcome is coded 0 = alive, 1 = dead;
diabetes is coded 1 = diabetic, 0 = non-diabetic
Select 'Analyze'
Select 'Survival'
Select 'Kaplan–Meier'
Move *months* to 'Time' box; *outcome* to 'Status' box;Select 'Define Event', next to 'Single value' put 1
Move *diabetes* to 'Factor' box
Select 'Options'and tick 'Survival table' under 'Statistics'
Select 'Compare factor' and tick'log rank' under'Test statistics'

Output given for every time point in the data. Most have been deleted from this output

Survival Analysis for months

Factor diab = diabetic

Time	Status	Cumulative Survival	Standard Error	Cumulative Events	Number Remaining
1.00000	1	.9583	.0408	1	23
1.10000	1	.9167	.0564	2	22
lines omitted					
10.03333	1	.7083	.0928	7	17
14.13333	0			7	16
lines omitted					
45.43333	1	.4482	.1118	12	7
59.63334	0			12	6
72.40000	1	.3735	.1155	13	5

Cumulative survival only shown where it changes. For points where it is blank use the one above

Number of Cases: 24   Censored: 10   (41.67%)   Events: 14

Factor diab = non-diabetic

Time	Status	Cumulative Survival	Standard Error	Cumulative Events	Number Remaining
.43333	1	.9884	.0116	1	85
.46667	1	.9767	.0163	2	84
lines omitted					
10.70000	1	.8820	.0351	10	74
13.53333	1	.8701	.0366	11	73
lines omitted					
56.03333	1	.5577	.0555	36	42
60.60000	1	.5444	.0557	37	41
62.23333	1	.5312	.0559	38	40

More concise output can be obtained from the **Life Tables** command but will calculate on grouped data

Number of Cases: 86   Censored: 39   (45.35%)   Events: 47

To calculate 95% confidence interval of survival rate use large sample Normal approximation.
Limits are cumulative survival ± 1.96 × standard error.
For non-diabetics at 60 months this is 0.5577 ± 1.96 × 0.0555, i.e. 0.4489 to 0.6665 or 45% to 67%.

Survival Analysis for months

		Total	Number Events	Number Censored	Percent Censored
diab	diabetic	24	14	10	41.67
diab	non-diabetic	86	47	39	45.35
Overall		110	61	49	44.55

Test Statistics for Equality of Survival Distributions for diab

	Statistic	df	Significance
Log Rank	1.74	1	.1867

P value for log rank test

Figure 11.5 Output for Kaplan–Meier estimates of survival and log rank test in SPSS

11.3 The log rank test

It is possible to compare survival curves by comparing the survival at a particular point. However, this causes some difficulty since there are many different points that could be chosen and the choice is arbitrary. To test the difference in the curves at several points would lead to multiple testing and spurious significance. The log rank test avoids this problem by comparing the whole of the curve for each of the groups.

The log rank test makes no assumptions about the shape of the survival curves provided that they do not cross. If they do cross, the survival experiences may be still be different, although there may be no overall tendency for one group to have better or worse survival. For example, in a cancer trial one group may experience early deaths due to drug toxicity but have better long-term survival. In this case we cannot say that one drug has better or worse death rates overall and different time periods need to be investigated separately.

The test is summarised in Box 11.5. Several books contain worked examples of this test (Altman *et al.* 2000; Swinscow and Campbell 2002). Figures 11.4 and 11.5 show the Stata and SPSS outputs for this test, and it is included in the reporting of the analysis in Box 11.4.

11.4 Cox regression

Previously we have compared survival in two or more groups using the log rank test. We have also calculated estimates of survival at specific points to allow the curves to be directly compared. However, it would be useful to have an overall measure of comparison of the survival experience of the groups. This can be done using the hazard ratio which is calculated using the Cox proportional hazards model. The hazard ratio is the ratio of the probability or risk of an event occurring in one group compared with another, and the interpretation is similar to a relative risk. (The hazard ratio is sometimes referred to as a relative risk, but is more correctly called the hazard ratio.)

There are no assumptions about the shape of the survival curve, but the method assumes that the ratio of the probability of an event taking place in the two groups does not change over time. The simplest way to check this assumption is to look at the survival curves. In small datasets there may be some crossing over of curves if the curves are close together even if the assumption holds.

Box 11.6 summarises the method and its assumptions. For further discussion of methods to check the assumptions, see Campbell (2001) or Kirkwood and

months is the follow-up time in months
outcome is coded 0 = alive, 1 = dead
diabetes is coded 1 = diabetic, 0 = non-diabetic

stset describes the survival variables in the data (see Figure 11.1)

```
. stset months, failure(outcome)
```

output omitted but same as in figure 11.1

```
. stcox diabetes

         failure _d:  outcome
   analysis time _t:  months

Iteration 0:   log likelihood =  -256.5776
Iteration 1:   log likelihood = -255.79451
Iteration 2:   log likelihood = -255.77879
Iteration 3:   log likelihood = -255.77879
Refining estimates:
Iteration 0:   log likelihood = -255.77879

Cox regression -- Breslow method for ties

No. of subjects =           110          Number of obs   =        110
No. of failures =            61
Time at risk    =   5617.866647
                                         LR chi2(1)      =       1.60
Log likelihood  =    -255.77879          Prob > chi2     =     0.2062

------------------------------------------------------------------------
     _t | Haz. Ratio   Std. Err.      z    P>|z|    [95% Conf. Interval]
--------+---------------------------------------------------------------
diabetes |   1.493624   .4568792    1.31   0.190    .8201068    2.720272
------------------------------------------------------------------------
```

Hazard ratio and 95% confidence interval   *P* value for hypothesis that hazard ratio is 1

Figure 11.6 Output for Cox regression with one predictor variable in Stata

Sterne (2003). We suggest that researchers seek the advice of a statistician when analysing survival data as it a complex procedure to perform and interpret.

11.4.1 Presenting the results of the single variable Cox regression

Figures 11.6 and 11.7 show the outputs from Stata and SPSS for the single variable Cox regression analysis. The analysis is carried out on the logarithm of the hazard ratio. SPSS gives the regression coefficients, referred to as B. The hazard ratio, referred to as exp(B), and the confidence interval for the hazard ratio need to be requested in the options. Box 11.7 shows how the results of this Cox regression analysis can be presented as an addition to the analysis presented earlier in Box 11.4.

BOX 11.7 EXAMPLE

Presenting Cox regression with one predictor variable

Peripheral vascular disease study

(*This adds to the analysis and description in Box 11.4*).

Methods section

Cox regression was used to calculate the hazard ratio and 95% confidence interval.

Results section

Diabetics had shorter survival time than non-diabetics, but this was not significant (hazard ratio 1.49, 95% CI 0.82 to 2.72, $P = 0.190$).

months is the follow-up time in months
outcome is coded 0 = alive, 1 = dead
diabetes is coded 1 = diabetic, 0 = non-diabetic
Select 'Analyze'
Select 'Survival'
Select 'Cox regression'
Move *months* to 'Time' box; *outcome* to 'Status' box; Select 'Define Event', next to 'Single value' put '1'
Move *diabetes* to 'Covariates' box
Select 'Options' and tick 'CI for Exp(B)'

Cox Regression

Case Processing Summary

		N	Percent	
Cases available in analysis	Event(a)	61	50.4%	
	Censored	49	40.5%	Check the numbers here are as expected: 61 have died out of a total of 110; 11 subjects had missing follow-up times
	Total	110	90.9%	
Cases dropped	Cases with missing values	11	9.1%	
	Cases with negative time	0	.0%	
	Censored cases before the earliest event in a stratum	0	.0%	
	Total	11	9.1%	
Total		121	100.0%	

a Dependent Variable: months

Block 0: Beginning Block
Omnibus Tests of Model Coefficients
Table omitted

Block 1: Method = Enter
Omnibus Tests of Model Coefficients(a,b)
Table omitted

Variables in the Equation

	B	SE	Wald	df	Sig.	Exp(B)	95.0% CI for Exp(B)	
							Lower	Upper
diabetes	.401	.306	1.720	1	.190	1.494	.820	2.720

Covariate Means

	Mean
diabetes	.218

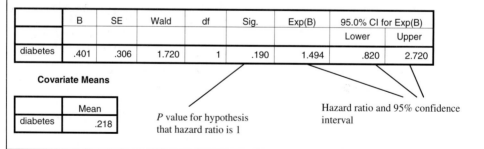

P value for hypothesis that hazard ratio is 1

Hazard ratio and 95% confidence interval

Figure 11.7 Output for Cox regression with one predictor variable in SPSS

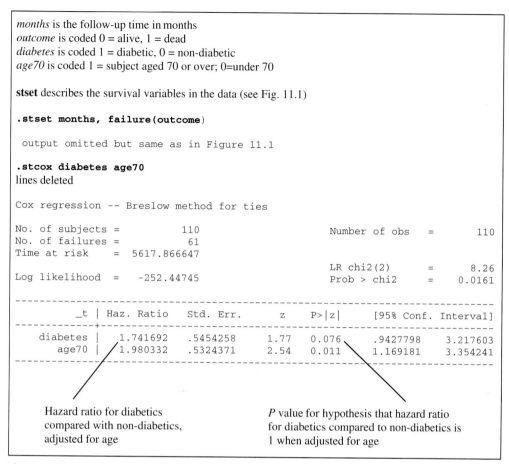

months is the follow-up time in months
outcome is coded 0 = alive, 1 = dead
diabetes is coded 1 = diabetic, 0 = non-diabetic
age70 is coded 1 = subject aged 70 or over; 0=under 70

stset describes the survival variables in the data (see Fig. 11.1)

```
.stset months, failure(outcome)
```

```
 output omitted but same as in Figure 11.1
```

```
.stcox diabetes age70
```
lines deleted

```
Cox regression -- Breslow method for ties

No. of subjects =          110                 Number of obs   =          110
No. of failures =           61
Time at risk    =   5617.866647
                                               LR chi2(2)      =         8.26
Log likelihood  =    -252.44745                Prob > chi2     =       0.0161

------------------------------------------------------------------------------
         _t |  Haz. Ratio   Std. Err.      z    P>|z|     [95% Conf. Interval]
------------+-----------------------------------------------------------------
    diabetes |   1.741692    .5454258     1.77   0.076     .9427798    3.217603
      age70 |   1.980332    .5324371     2.54   0.011     1.169181    3.354241
------------------------------------------------------------------------------
```

Hazard ratio for diabetics
compared with non-diabetics,
adjusted for age

P value for hypothesis that hazard ratio
for diabetics compared to non-diabetics is
1 when adjusted for age

Figure 11.8 Output for Cox regression with more than one predictor variable in Stata

11.4.2 Comment on the results

It was noted that age was significantly related to the risk of death and may be an important confounder in assessing the contribution of other risk factors. The diabetic subjects were younger than the non-diabetics, and so might be expected to have a lower death rate. The difference in age between the diabetics and non-diabetics might have reduced the estimated effect of diabetes on peripheral vascular disease that was seen in the survival curves.

11.4.3 Extending the analysis

In the previous section we used Cox regression to perform an analysis with just one predictor variable. However, Cox regression can be used to fit multifactorial models with several predictor variables and therefore can be used to estimate the hazard ratios after adjusting for other variables. Therefore we extended the analysis to adjust for age. The Stata and SPSS outputs are shown in Figures 11.8 and 11.9.

The unadjusted and the adjusted hazard ratios are shown in the table in Box 11.8. The adjusted hazard ratio for diabetes is larger than the unadjusted ratio, but the confidence interval still crosses 1. The Kaplan–Meier survival curve has not been repeated here, but is referred to in the text and should be included where possible for the main comparison of interest.

Note that it is possible to adjust Kaplan–Meier curves in Stata, which would show the curves to be further apart than in Box 11.4 (Missouris *et al.* 2004).

months is the follow-up time in months
outcome is coded 0 = alive, 1 = dead
diabetes is coded 1 = diabetic, 0 = non-diabetic
age70 is coded 1 = subject aged 70 or over; 0=under 70
Select 'Analyze'
Select 'Survival'
Select 'Cox regression'
Move *months* to 'Time' box; *outcome* to 'Status' box; Select 'Define Event', next to 'Single value' put 1
Move *diabetes, age70* to 'Covariates' box
Select 'Options' and tick 'CI for Exp(B)'

Cox Regression
Case Processing Summary
Table same as in Figure 11.6

Block 0: Beginning Block
Omnibus Tests of Model Coefficients
Table omitted

Block 1: Method = Enter
Omnibus Tests of Model Coefficients(a,b)
Table omitted

Variables in the Equation

	B	SE	Wald	df	Sig.	Exp(B)	95.0% CI for Exp(B)	
							Lower	Upper
diabetes	.555	.313	3.139	1	.076	1.742	.942	3.218
age70	.683	.269	6.458	1	.011	1.980	1.169	3.354

Covariate Means
Table omitted

P value for hypothesis that hazard ratio for diabetics compared with non-diabetics is 1, when adjusted for age

Hazard ratio and 95% confidence interval for diabetics compared with non diabetics, adjusted for age

Figure 11.9 Output for Cox regression with more than one predictor variable in SPSS

BOX 11.8 EXAMPLE

Presenting Cox regression analysis

Peripheral vascular disease study

Aim of study To assess the long term survival of patients with peripheral vascular disease (PVD) and to investigate the impact of the presence of risk factors on mortality.

Study design Cohort study.

Patient population Consecutive patients with PVD and intermittent claudication who were referred for angiography and found to have angiographic evidence of PVD.

Aim of analysis To compare survival rates in those with and without risk factors, including diabetes.

Table. Survival rates and hazard ratios for risk factors of mortality in patients with PVD

Risk factor		Number of deaths (%)	Percentage surviving 5 years	Hazard ratio (95% CI)	Hazard ratio adjusted for age (95% CI)
Age	≥70	37 (64)	38 (26 to 51)	1.83 (1.09 to 3.06)	
	<70	24 (46)	69 (54 to 80)		
Diabetes	Yes	14 (58)	45 (23 to 65)	1.49 (0.82 to 2.72)	1.74 (0.94 to 3.22)
	No	47 (55)	56 (44 to 66)		

Description

Methods section

Survival rates are expressed as the percentage surviving for 5 years calculated using the Kaplan–Meier method. Cox proportional hazards was used to calculate the hazard ratios and 95% confidence intervals for risk factors. Age was treated as a covariate. All analysis was carried out in Stata version 8.

Results section

A total of 110 patients were included in this analysis. Mean follow-up time of survivors was 6.1 years; range 14 days to 8.7 years. Thirty-five men and 26 women (55%) died. The Kaplan–Meier curve shows that patients with diabetes have lower survival rates (Box 11.4). The log rank test gave $P = 0.19$.

The risk of mortality was nearly twofold in patients over 70 compared with those under 70. After adjusting for age, patients with diabetes had an increased risk of mortality compared with non-diabetics, but this was not significant (table). Further adjustment for sex was made but had little effect on the hazard ratio (hazard ratio 1.70; 95% CI (0.96 to 3.37, $P = 0.069$).

11.5 Further reading

The references given in Box 11.9 are those that we have found particularly useful for the specific topics listed.

BOX 11.9 INFORMATION

Useful references to statistical details presented in this chapter

Introductory accounts

Bland 2000 chapter 15, Altman *et al.* 2000 chapter 4, Campbell 2001, Swinscow and Campbell 2002

Survival plots

Pocock *et al.* 2002

Assumptions

Bland 2000 chapter 15

When assumptions do not hold

Kirkwood and Sterne 2003

Fuller accounts

Altman 1991 chapter 13, Armitage *et al.* 2002 chapter 17, Parmar and Machin1995, Campbell 2001

Worked examples of the Kaplan–Meier methods

Altman *et al.* 2000 chapter 4, Swinscow and Cambell 2002

Chapter summary

Survival analysis

- Survival methods are used to analyse time-to-event data. The outcome is not always death; for example, it can be time to recurrence, time to miscarriage, time to conception, etc.
- Present the number of events, follow-up time, and variability in follow-up time
- Describe any censored observations and justify any assumptions made about them
- Survival curves should be shown, indicating censoring or numbers at risk
- Beware of imprecision in the right-hand side of the survival curve
- Estimate survival probabilities at a fixed time point, with 95% confidence intervals, using a method which takes into account censored observations (e.g. Kaplan–Meier)
- Beware of comparing survival at several points along the curves unless there is a strong prior hypothesis, as this is multiple hypothesis testing and may lead to spurious significant results
- Use the log rank test to provide an overall comparison of two or more curves
- Present the hazard ratio with a 95% CI to estimate the difference in survival between two groups of interest. This can be calculated using Cox regression
- Use Cox regression to adjust survival for several variables
- Check that the assumptions for Cox regression hold

CHAPTER 12

Presenting a randomised controlled trial

12.1 Introduction to the CONSORT statement

In the 1990s an international group of clinical trialists, statisticians, epidemiologists, and editors developed the CONSORT statement (**Con**solidated **S**tandards **o**f **R**eporting **T**rials) to guide researchers on the reporting of randomised controlled trials (Begg *et al.* 1996). The CONSORT statement comprises a checklist and diagram, and explanatory notes, and was revised and expanded in 2001 (Altman *et al.* 2001; Moher *et al.* 2001). Now CONSORT has been adopted by many biomedical editors as the standard for submissions to their journals and the guidelines are readily available on the web (www.consort-statement.org). We summarise the rationale behind CONSORT in Box 12.1.

The CONSORT checklist is shown in Box 12.2. Detailed explanatory notes, with examples of good practice, are given on the CONSORT website and are well worth reading. The guidelines were designed for trials where individuals are randomly allocated to one of two or more treatment groups. However, the principles clearly apply to other more complex experimental designs.

In this chapter we will give examples of using the CONSORT statement to guide the presentation of statistical aspects of a two group trial with individual randomisation. We will give examples from trials published in papers.

The same principles of reporting apply when presenting a trial in a longer document where space is less restricted and the researcher is able to report in more detail than is possible in most journal

BOX 12.1 INFORMATION

The CONSORT Statement

Background

◆ Evidence-based medicine requires reliable scientific information about what are effective health care interventions

◆ Randomised controlled trials which are rigorously designed and carefully conducted provide the best evidence for effective interventions

◆ The quality of the design and reporting of randomised trials is known to be variable

◆ Flaws in design and reporting have been associated with biased and unreliable results

CONSORT

◆ **Con**solidated **S**tandards **o**f **R**eporting **T**rials

◆ 22-item checklist and flowchart template, with accompanying explanatory notes

◆ Provides a common standard of reporting of trials to guide researchers in presenting randomised trials

◆ Provides a framework for the critical review of randomised trials to facilitate valid decisions about health care practice

BOX 12.2 INFORMATION

CONSORT checklist (www.consort-statement.org)

	Item number	Descriptor
Title and abstract	1	How participants were allocated to interventions (e.g. 'random allocation', 'randomised', or 'randomly assigned')
Introduction		
Background	2	Scientific background and explanation of rationale
Methods		
Participants	3	Eligibility criteria for participants and the settings and locations where the data were collected
Interventions	4	Precise details of the interventions intended for each group and how and when they were actually administered
Objectives	5	Specific objectives and hypotheses
Outcomes	6	Clearly defined primary and secondary outcome measures and, when applicable, any methods used to enhance the quality of measurements (e.g. multiple observations, training of assessors, etc.)
Sample size	7	How sample size was determined and, when applicable, explanation of any interim analyses and stopping rules
Randomisation sequence generation	8	Method used to generate the random allocation sequence, including details of any restriction (e.g. blocking, stratification)
Allocation concealment	9	Method used to implement the random allocation sequence (e.g. numbered containers or central telephone), clarifying whether the sequence was concealed until interventions were assigned.

BOX 12.2 *(Continued)*

CONSORT checklist (www.consort-statement.org)

	Item number	Descriptor
Implementation	10	Who generated the allocation sequence, who enrolled the participants, and who assigned participants to their groups.
Blinding (masking)	11	Whether or not participants, those administering the interventions, and those assessing the outcomes were aware of group assignment; if not, how the success of masking was assessed
Statistical methods	12	Statistical method used to compare groups for primary outcome(s); methods for additional analyses, such as subgroup analyses and adjusted analyses.
Results		
Participant flow	13	Flow of participants through each stage (a diagram is strongly recommended). Specifically, for each group report the numbers of participants randomly assigned, receiving intended treatment, completing the study protocol, and analysed for the primary outcome. Describe protocol deviations from study as planned, together with reasons
Recruitment	14	Dates defining the periods of recruitment and follow-up
Baseline data	15	Baseline demographic and clinical characteristics of each group
Numbers analysed	16	Number of participants (denominator) in each group included in each analysis and whether the analysis was by 'intention to treat'. State the results in absolute numbers when feasible (e.g. 10/20, not 50%)
Outcomes and estimation	17	For each primary and secondary outcome, a summary of results for each group, and the estimated effect size and its precision (e.g. 95% confidence interval)
Ancillary analyses	18	Address multiplicity by reporting any other analyses performed including subgroup analyses and adjusted analyses, indicating those pre-specified and those exploratory
Adverse events	19	All important adverse events or side effects in each intervention group
Discussion		
Interpretation	20	Interpretation of the results, taking into account study hypotheses, sources of potential bias or imprecision, and the dangers associated with multiplicity of analyses and outcomes
Generalisability	21	Generalisability (external validity) of the trial findings
Overall evidence	22	General interpretation of the results in the context of current evidence

articles. (Web publishing now means that some journals publish a shorter version of articles on paper and a fuller version on the web, and so space is becoming less of an issue.) At the conclusion of the chapter, we will briefly mention other designs, such as cluster designs, and summarise additional guidelines for reporting them.

12.2 The CONSORT checklist

We will focus attention on the reporting of items which relate to Statistics and will refer back to previous sections in the book where an issue has been discussed before. We will indicate the CONSORT checklist items discussed in each paragraph.

Examples for CONSORT checklist items relating to the trial methods

Item 1

Title

'High-frequency oscillatory ventilation for the prevention of chronic lung disease of prematurity'

Allocation to intervention (Abstract)

'We randomly assigned preterm infants with a gestational age of 23 to 28 weeks to either conventional or high-frequency oscillatory ventilation . . .'

Item 3

Eligibility criteria

'Infants were eligible for the study if their gestational age was between 23 weeks and 28 weeks plus 6 days; if they were born in a participating centre; if they required endotracheal intubation from birth; and if they required ongoing intensive care. Infants were excluded if they had to be transferred to another hospital for intensive care shortly after birth or if they had a major congenital malformation.'

Settings and locations

'A total of 25 centres participated in the study—22 in the United Kingdom and 1 each in Australia, Ireland, and Singapore. To ensure that each centre had adequate experience with high-frequency oscillatory ventilation, we required participating centres to have used this type of ventilatory support in a minimum of 20 infants before the study began.'

Item 6

Outcomes

'The primary outcome measure was a composite of death or chronic lung disease (defined by a dependence on supplemental oxygen) at 36 weeks of postmenstrual age. Secondary outcome measures were age at death, age at hospital discharge, major abnormality on cranial ultrasonography, air leak, failure of treatment, failure on hearing testing, necrotising enterocolitis, patent ductus arteriosus requiring treatment, treatment with postnatal systemic corticosteroids, pulmonary haemorrhage, and retinopathy of prematurity.'

Item 7

Sample size

'A sample size of 800 to 1200 infants was needed, given the assumption that 30% of the study population would have a gestational age of 23 to 25 weeks and 70% would have a gestational age of 26 to 28 weeks and that the incidence of the primary outcome would be 75% for the lower gestational age group and 48% for the higher gestational age group. With a sample of this size, the study had 90% power (at a significance level 0.05), to detect a difference between treatment groups of 9 to 11 percentage points.'

Items 8–10

Randomisation

'Infants were randomised in blocks of four to either conventional ventilation or high frequency oscillatory ventilation, with stratification according to gestational age (two strata) and according to centre (25 strata).'

Item 12

Statistical methods

'An independent committee reviewed statistical analyses performed at 12 and 18 months after recruitment began and found no reason to stop the trial early. P values (*for the primary outcome*) were adjusted to preserve an overall level of significance as 0.05. For the secondary outcomes (both main effects and interactions), we used the Bonferroni method to correct for multiple testing, which resulted in the use of a P value of 0.004 to indicate significance. All reported P values are uncorrected unless otherwise stated.'

BOX 12.3 *(Continued)*

'Unadjusted relative risks or hazard ratios, as appropriate, with 95% confidence intervals, were calculated to estimate the relative effect of high-frequency oscillatory ventilation as compared with that of conventional ventilation for all outcomes. Logistic regression or Cox regression was used to investigate treatment effects with gestational age (23 to 25 weeks or 26 to 28 weeks) and location (United Kingdom and Ireland; Australia; or Singapore) as covariates. Interaction terms were fitted in the model in order to assess differences in treatment effects according to gestational age and location. Baseline variables with the potential to be important prognostic factors were identified in advance of the analysis. We decided to include them in the model only if a clinically important imbalance was observed. All statistical analyses were performed according to the intention-to-treat principle, with the use of Stata software.'

(Johnson *et al.* 2002)

12.2.1 Title and abstract (checklist item 1)

The title of the paper and/or the abstract should indicate that the study is a randomised trial so that it is indexed by electronic databases as a trial, and is thus accessible to other researchers performing electronic searches. Journals have different policies about titles. Some journals insist that the study design is included as part of the title of the paper, but other journals have a tight word limit for the title which may make it difficult to do this.

In UKOS, the title did not mention 'trial' or 'randomised' or similar, but it was clear from the abstract that this was a trial (Box 12.3).

12.2.2 Participants (checklist item 3)

The report should state the inclusion and exclusion criteria, and the settings and locations of the trial. These factors are important because they assist the interpretation of the trial results, and indicate the participant group to which the findings can be generalised.

An example is shown in Box 12.3. Note that there were eligibility criteria for the centres, as well as inclusion criteria for the participants within the centres.

12.2.3 Intervention (checklist item 4)

For any trial the interventions need to be clearly defined, including what steps were taken to disguise a placebo. However, in non-drug trials some detailed explanation may be required to describe the different components of the intervention. In a review of six trials of nurse-led hypertension clinics (Oakeshott *et al.* 2005), some trials had allowed the nurse to prescribe or recommend changes in drug treatment, while in others the emphasis was on healthy lifestyle advice. This highlights the need to describe the exact details of the intervention, and also to define what is meant by 'usual care'. In addition, it may be important to report how the people were selected to administer the intervention, and what training they received, for example in trials of acupuncture or physical therapy (UK BEAM 2004).

12.2.4 Outcomes (checklist item 6)

The researcher should first state which is the primary outcome, and then any secondary outcomes. The primary outcome is the endpoint which will be used to determine if there is a real difference between the two interventions, and is used in the sample size calculations. Secondary outcomes are other outcomes of interest, and may include adverse effects of the interventions. For each outcome, but especially the primary outcome, the type of data should be clear. For example, is it a measurement or a score or a category? This information helps the reader to understand the statistical analysis, and it aids the interpretation of the findings.

In the example (Box 12.3), we have reported the primary outcome and secondary outcomes. We have defined terms which are potentially ambiguous or uncommon such as 'chronic lung disease'. The primary outcome is a yes/no (binary) variable.

12.2.5 Sample size (checklist item 7)

The presentation of sample size follows the guidelines we have given in Chapter 3. It is important to give enough information to allow the calculations to be checked by reviewers and other researchers.

Information required is the power and significance level, and the difference between treatment groups (effect size) that can be detected with the target number of participants. For continuous variables, the standard deviation should be given. In addition, it is important to say if the comparisons will be two-tailed. One-tailed comparisons are rarely appropriate in trials and, if used, careful justification should be given. If the sample size calculations have made allowance for attrition during the trial, this should be described.

The clinically meaningful difference in treatments is important not only to allow the sample size calculations to be checked, but also to aid interpretation of the observed difference in treatment groups. Some studies report expected differences which are very large and which seem implausible. This can arise if the researcher's baseline (control group) estimate is too low and/or the anticipated estimate (intervention group) is too high. Sometimes, large 'expected' treatment differences result from the researcher having a small fixed available sample size, and so he/she has 'worked backwards' to calculate the difference which this sample size could detect. In this situation, the trial is very likely to produce a smaller difference in treatment outcome than expected. This will be non-significant and therefore the trial will be inconclusive.

The statement from UKOS is shown in Box 12.3. Two things are worth noting here. First, a range was given for the target sample size. This represented minimum and maximum feasible numbers which could be recruited in the time available and therefore translated into a range for the difference to be detected. The clinicians felt that this was reasonable since defining the clinically meaningful difference involves judgement. Secondly, two values were given for the estimated proportion with the primary outcome: one in the lower gestational age infants and the other in the higher gestational age infants. The calculations were presented in this way because it is common to present outcome rates for lower- and higher gestational age infants separately, and therefore this showed clearly how the overall figures were obtained.

Where trials have interim analyses for data monitoring purposes, it is important to state how many times the committee met and what steps were taken to deal with multiple testing of data monitoring outcomes. If a complex stopping rule was used, this should be described. The UKOS paper reported the data monitoring information with the other statistical analysis (Box 12.3, item 12). It is not always necessary to follow the checklist order if information fits better elsewhere. The important thing is to include all the information in a clear format.

12.2.6 Randomisation (checklist items 8–10)

The CONSORT checklist requires fairly detailed information on the randomisation process. This includes reporting how the random sequence was generated, confirming that it was truly random, and stating who allocated participants to their groups. For example, the trial might have used another department, which was not involved in the study, to determine the random sequence and inform the researcher which treatment a newly recruited participant should receive. Alternatively a telephone or web-based service could be used. It should be clear who has recruited the participants, since it is important to be able to demonstrate that the randomisation was separate from the recruitment and therefore that the recruitment of participants could not be biased by knowledge of the allocation sequence.

If unrestricted simple randomisation is used, this should be stated. If randomisation was restricted using blocks and/or strata, this should be described, stating the block size and listing the stratification variables.

The statement shown in Box 12.3 comes from the published paper and is noticeably brief. The original UKOS submission included details of the recruitment process and the telephone randomisation service, stating that the randomisation sequence was hidden from the clinicians until the participant was recruited and the telephone randomisation service was assured that the participant met the eligibility criteria. Unfortunately, these details had to be omitted in the final publication because of lack of space.

The checklist in Box 12.2 assumes that patients are individually randomised to intervention groups. If this is not the case, then the unit of randomisation should be stated. Section 12.4 describes the key features of cluster randomised designs where groups of individuals are randomised to intervention groups.

12.2.7 Blinding (checklist item 11)

Blinding is important to avoid biased assessment and should be reported when it is used. Researchers should report if the participants were blind to the treatment allocation, since knowledge of the treatment has been shown to affect a participant's response. It is also important to report whether those assessing the outcome were blinded to the treatment allocated since, again, knowledge of the treatment received by a participant may subconsciously or consciously affect the assessment of all outcomes, with the probable exception of death.

Trials are not always conducted blind, and in some cases blinding is impossible, for example when the interventions are two different technologies.

In UKOS the intervention was one of two types of ventilator which could not be concealed from the clinician. The participants in UKOS were infants and so would be unaware of the type of intervention. Wherever possible, assessments were done by independent observers who were unaware of the ventilator used. It may also be possible to choose methods of measurements which are more objective than alternatives. For example, the use of automatic blood pressure measuring devices may be less prone to observer bias than a mercury sphygmomanometer. It is important to report these design features since this increases the validity of the data.

12.2.8 **Statistical methods (checklist item 12)**

This section should document the type of analysis performed to compare the primary outcome between the two groups. Unless it is obvious, any assumptions of the methods should be justified. The researcher should describe the method used for any adjusted analyses, including the choice of variables to adjust for. Any subgroup analyses should also be described. Where adjustment was made for baseline imbalance, this should be described and justified. Any adjustment for multiple testing should be described. The researcher should say if analyses were performed according to the intention to treat, and if not, then this should be justified (see section 12.3.1). It is helpful to state the statistical program used for the analysis.

The UKOS statement in Box 12.3 includes details of most of these points. In particular, we described the methods used for adjustment for multiple testing, the methods for testing subgroup effects, and the strategy for dealing with imbalance in baseline variables.

12.2.9 **Participant flow and recruitment details (checklist items 13 and 14)**

There needs to be a complete audit trail of a trial so that all participants are accounted for. Details should be given of all eligible participants, with reasons for non-recruitment where available. Numbers of, and reasons for, post-randomisation losses should be documented. A diagram is often the best way to show the flow of participants from recruitment to analysis. Figure 12.1 shows the template from the CONSORT website. A Word version can be downloaded for use.

The UKOS diagram is shown in Figure 12.2. The diagram makes clear how many infants were eligible and how many of these were recruited, plus the reasons for non-recruitment. Since consent and randomisation sometimes happened before birth, some infants were later found to be ineligible and were excluded. Further losses occurred because of withdrawals for various reasons. All infants were accounted for, showing finally the number of infants included in the analysis of the primary outcome.

It is also important to report the dates of the trial. This is necessary since the date of publication of a paper may not be a good indicator of when the trial took place. In Figure 12.2 we also show how the recruitment process can be described in the text.

Any protocol deviations should be reported in the original randomisation groups.

12.2.10 **Baseline data (checklist item 15)**

It is important to present baseline data in a trial for two reasons. The first is to show the characteristics of the group to allow readers to judge the significance of the trial results to a specific individual. The second is to confirm that the two randomised groups are balanced for key prognostic variables. If the participants have been allocated to the two groups at random, then any imbalance between the groups must be due to chance alone, unless the randomisation process was faulty.

It is common practice to use a significance test to compare the two groups at baseline (pre-randomisation) and to report a P value for this. We do not recommend this practice for the following reason. If participants have been allocated randomly to the two groups, any differences between the groups must be due to chance alone. Hence testing against chance makes no sense.

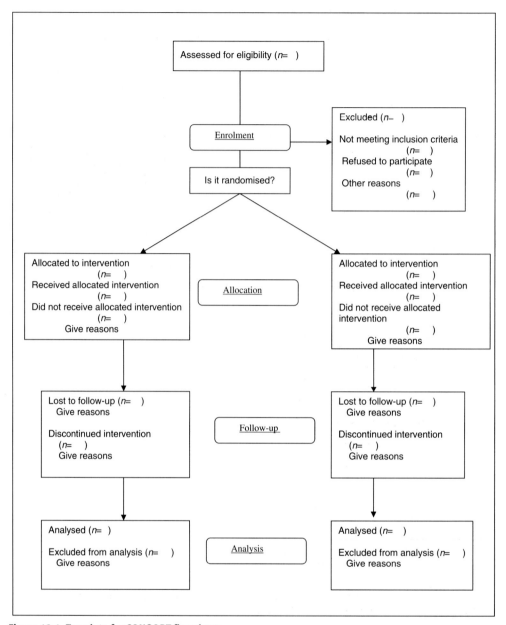

Figure 12.1 Template for CONSORT flowchart

In common with the reporting of descriptive data for a single group (Chapter 5), the baseline data table should include the following information for each group: number of subjects, the mean and standard deviation for continuous data, and the proportion or percentage with the numerator and denominator for categorical data.

In Box 12.4 we show an extract from one of the two tables of baseline variables from UKOS with a sentence describing these findings. (We presented baseline data for mothers and infants separately.) Note that data were incomplete for some variables. This is unfortunate and was due to missing data in the patients' medical notes.

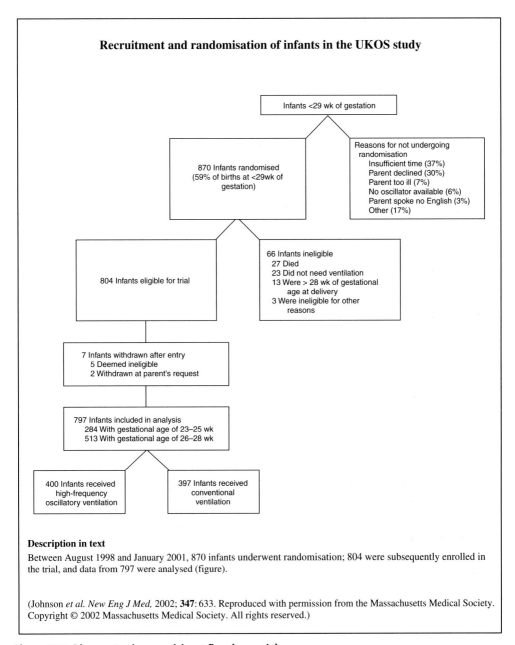

Recruitment and randomisation of infants in the UKOS study

Infants <29 wk of gestation

870 Infants randomised
(59% of births at <29wk of
gestation)

Reasons for not undergoing
randomisation
    Insufficient time (37%)
    Parent declined (30%)
    Parent too ill (7%)
    No oscillator available (6%)
    Parent spoke no English (3%)
    Other (17%)

66 Infants ineligible
    27 Died
    23 Did not need ventilation
    13 Were > 28 wk of gestational
        age at delivery
    3 Were ineligible for other
        reasons

804 Infants eligible for trial

7 Infants withdrawn after entry
    5 Deemed ineligible
    2 Withdrawn at parent's request

797 Infants included in analysis
    284 With gestational age of 23–25 wk
    513 With gestational age of 26–28 wk

400 Infants received
high-frequency
oscillatory ventilation

397 Infants received
conventional
ventilation

Description in text

Between August 1998 and January 2001, 870 infants underwent randomisation; 804 were subsequently enrolled in the trial, and data from 797 were analysed (figure).

(Johnson *et al. New Eng J Med,* 2002; **347**:633. Reproduced with permission from the Massachusetts Medical Society. Copyright © 2002 Massachusetts Medical Society. All rights reserved.)

Figure 12.2 Diagram to show participant flow (example)

BOX 12.4 EXAMPLE

Example for CONSORT checklist item relating to baseline variables

Table. Baseline characteristics of the mother (extract)

Characteristic	High-frequency oscillatory ventilation N=364	Conventional ventilation N=353
Age (yr) (mean (SD))	29 (6.4)	29 (6.1)
Race (no./total (%))		
White	290/363 (80)	276/353 (78)
Black	35/363 (10)	31/353 (9)
Other	38/363 (10)	46/353 (13)
Pre-existing or pregnancy-induced diabetes	11/364 (3)	7/351 (2)
Smoking in pregnancy (no./total (%))	95/334 (28)	86/321 (27)
Caesarean section		
After labour	75/364 (21)	64/353 (18)
Without labour	134/364 (37)	125/353 (35)

Note: the total numbers relate to mothers not infants as some births were multiple.

Description

The two treatment groups were well balanced for maternal characteristics (table).

(Johnson *et al.* 2002)

12.2.11 Outcome data (checklist item 17)

Since the primary outcome is the endpoint used to assess the effectiveness of the two study interventions, it is essential that it is prominently reported in the text and in the abstract, whatever the results may show. All specified secondary outcomes should similarly also be reported, whether significant or not. For all outcomes the effect size should be given with a measure of precision, such as a confidence interval, except where this is not possible, for example when using rank-based methods. If there is space, the P value could be given as well. Findings should never be presented in terms of a P value alone without any estimate of the size of difference and its precision.

These guidelines should be followed whether or not the primary or secondary outcome is statistically significant. Confidence intervals are especially important where a finding is not statistically significant since it will indicate whether an important clinical difference is possible.

It is quite common to present a confidence interval for each group separately. This is not helpful since we are mainly interested in the difference between the groups and we cannot easily deduce that from two separate intervals. Also, reporting two separate intervals plus an interval for the difference clutters the results.

In Box 12.5 we show an extract of the outcome data for UKOS and the wording used to describe the findings. The primary outcome was binary and the difference between the two ventilation groups was expressed as a relative risk with a 95% confidence interval. The difference between the two treatment groups was small (two percentage points); the interval spanned 1.0 and was clearly not significant. Had the difference been significant, we might have chosen to calculate the number

BOX 12.5 EXAMPLE

Example for CONSORT checklist item relating to outcomes

Table. Primary and secondary outcomes at 36 weeks postmenstrual age (extract)

Outcome	High-frequency oscillatory ventilation	Conventional ventilation	Relative risk (HFOV/CV) (95% CI)
Primary outcome (no./total (%))			
All infants	265/400 (66)	268/397 (68)	0.98 (0.89 to 1.08)
Dead	100/400 (25)	105/397 (26)	
Alive, with chronic lung disease	165/400 (41)	163/397 (41)	
Alive, without chronic lung disease	135/400 (34)	129/397 (32)	
Secondary outcomes (no./total (%))			
Failure of treatment	41/400 (10)	41/397 (10)	0.99 (0.66 to 1.50)
Major cerebral abnormality	54/393 (14)	75/393 (19)	0.72 (0.52 to 0.99)
Air leak	64/399 (16)	72/395 (18)	0.88 (0.65 to 1.20)
Pulmonary haemorrhage	44/395 (11)	55/390 (14)	0.79 (0.55 to 1.14)

Description

The composite primary outcome of death or chronic lung disease (defined as dependence on supplementary oxygen) at 36 weeks of post-menstrual age occurred in 66% of infants assigned to high-frequency oscillatory ventilation and 68% of those assigned to conventional ventilation ($P = 0.71$) (table). Similar proportions of infants died (25% of those receiving high-frequency oscillatory ventilation vs 26% of those receiving conventional ventilation) or had chronic lung disease (41% in each group). . . . The proportions of infants with each of the specified secondary outcomes were also similar in the two groups (table). In particular, criteria for treatment failure were met in 10% of the infants in each group.

(Johnson *et al.* 2002)

needed to treat (see section 12.3.2) as well as the relative risk.

Note that the secondary outcome, major cerebral abnormality, has a 95% confidence interval that excludes 1.00 and so indicates significance at the 0.05 level. However, for secondary outcomes, the trial calculated a modified cut-off for significance (0.004) to avoid obtaining spurious significant results simply because of testing multiple variables. This was commented on in the discussion section of the paper. Note that if a Bonferroni correction is used for a set of significance tests, then the test becomes a test of the composite hypothesis.

12.2.12 Interpretation and presentation of a non-significant result (checklist item 20)

In describing the difference between the two treatment groups, it is important to interpret 'not significant' correctly. If the study is powered to detect a small clinically important difference, then a non-significant finding will indicate that there is no important difference between the groups. However, it does **not** mean that there is evidence for no difference at all, and it is essential to present the estimated difference between the groups and a confidence interval.

If the result is non-significant and the trial is small, then it is entirely possible that an important difference does exist but that the trial is simply too small to demonstrate this conclusively. It is always wrong to interpret non-significance as meaning that there is no difference between the treatments. As previously, the results should be presented with an estimated difference and confidence interval, and the description should state that the findings are inconclusive. The interpretation should centre on the confidence interval as indicating the possible range of values for the clinical difference.

Non-significant results should always be reported in both large and small trials. This allows the reader to interpret the findings in the light of other studies, and perhaps pool results with those of others in a meta-analysis to obtain a more precise overall estimate.

12.2.13 Ancillary analyses (checklist item 18)

Trialists sometimes perform other analyses which are not the primary or secondary outcome analyses described previously. Subgroup analyses fall into this category. Effects in subgroups should always be tested by fitting an interaction term in the model. For example, in UKOS we tested the effect of treatment in the two gestational age groups not by looking at the two groups separately, but by fitting an interaction term 'treatment $\times$ gestational age' in the model.

Subgroup analyses are often data driven, i.e. the idea of doing the analysis comes from looking at the data. This is problematic because if we observe a large effect and then test it, it is clearly more likely to be statistically significant than if we tested an observed effect that was small. Data-driven analyses are also known as post-hoc analyses and are best avoided. If they are done for exploratory reasons, then the findings should be clearly presented as exploratory and they should be cautiously interpreted.

12.3 Intention to treat analysis

12.3.1 Introduction

When subjects are randomised, the two groups should be comparable with respect to baseline characteristics. If any subjects are excluded after randomisation, this comparability will be compromised. This underlies the recommendation to carry out an intention to treat analysis where all subjects are analysed according to the groups to which they were originally allocated (section 12.2.8).

However, full application of intention to treat is only possible when complete outcome data are available for all subjects (Hollis and Campbell 1999). In many trials, subjects will have missing observations and these may not be a random sample of all subjects. It may be that patients who do not perceive any benefit from the intervention withdraw from the trial. In smoking cessation trials it is common practice to assume that patients who

drop out or do not give samples have continued to smoke (Bolliger *et al.* 2000) (Box 12.6). Such an approach would not be suitable for all trials, especially those with continuous outcomes (Hollis and Campbell 1999). Therefore it is important to describe clearly what steps have been taken to investigate any potential influence of missing responses.

Where patients have swapped treatment group, either by dropping out of active treatment or being given a different treatment, intention to treat

---

BOX 12.6 EXAMPLE

Example of intention to treat and numbers needed to treat (NNT)

Effects of oral nicotine inhalers on amount smoked

Aim of study To see if oral nicotine inhalers can result in long-term reduction in smoking.

Design Double blind randomised placebo-controlled trial.

Setting Two university hospital pulmonary clinics in Switzerland.

Participants 400 healthy volunteers willing to reduce their smoking but unable or unwilling to stop smoking immediately.

Intention to treat analysis

All patients were analysed according to original allocation. Patients who withdrew or were lost to follow up were assumed to have continued smoking.

Results

152/200 participants in the placebo group and 166/200 in the control group completed 4 months of follow up.

52 (26%) subjects in the active group stopped smoking.
18 (9%) subjects in the placebo group stopped smoking.

Risk difference was 0.17 (95% CI, 0.10 to 0.24).

Number needed to treat = 1 / (risk difference)
$$= 5.9 \ (95\% \ \text{CI}, \ 4.1 \ \text{to} \ 10.3)$$

(Bolliger *et al.* 2000)

analysis will tend to underestimate the treatment benefit. This may not be desirable in an equivalence trial and may be a reason for not carrying out an intention to treat analysis.

12.3.2 **Number needed to treat**

The number needed to treat (NNT) is the number of patients that we would need to treat with the new treatment to achieve one more success than with the old treatment. It is applicable only to binary outcomes, and the main features are presented in Box 12.7. It is the reciprocal of the risk difference, which needs to be calculated first, along with its 95% confidence interval. An example is shown in Box 12.6.

BOX 12.7 SUMMARY

Number needed to treat

- Used with binary outcomes
- Number needed to treat is the reciprocal of the risk difference (Box 7.9)
- Calculate the risk difference and 95% confidence interval and then take reciprocal of values
- Lowest possible value is 1 (negative values can be considered as the numbers needed to harm)
- Highest possible value is infinity (denoted by ∞)
- If confidence interval for risk difference spans 0 (e.g. $-p_L$ to p_U) then NNT can be written as $-\infty$ to $-1/p_L$, $1/p_U$ to ∞. It should not be written as $-1/p_L$ to $1/p_U$ (Bland 2000).
- Should only be used as an additional descriptive summary of result, not the main outcome presentation

---

If the results are not significant, the presentation is problematic as the confidence interval is not continuous and needs to be presented in two parts. For fuller discussion see Bland (2000).

12.4 **Cluster-randomised trials**

12.4.1 **Introduction**

Cluster-randomised trials are trials where groups of individuals, the clusters, are jointly allocated to an intervention so that all individuals within a cluster receive the same intervention. Cluster trials are commonly used in primary care research where it may be more practical to assign a whole general practice to the same intervention rather than to allocate individuals separately within a practice. Other units of randomisation have been used, such as hospital wards, schools, whole communities such as villages in developing countries, time periods (e.g. weeks), and airline flights.

Randomising clusters rather than individuals has consequences for the required sample size and the statistical analysis of a trial and therefore affects the presentation of a trial.

In general, the required sample size is greater when clusters are randomised because of the interdependence between individuals within each cluster. We summarise these points in Box 12.8. Methods for sample size calculations are shown in Kerry and Bland (1998a), and a simple way of analysing cluster-randomised trials using summary measures for each cluster is described in Kerry and Bland (1998b). For a fuller discussion of cluster trials, see the book by Donner and Klar (2000).

Campbell *et al.* (2004) proposed an extension to the CONSORT statement specifically for cluster trials. Like the general CONSORT statement, the statement for cluster trials provides explanations and examples of good practice. We summarise the main points in Box 12.9. Researchers conducting and reporting cluster trials will find the full document very helpful (available on CONSORT website).

12.4.2 **Recruitment bias**

In cluster-randomised trials extra care needs to be taken in reporting how the subjects within the clusters were identified and recruited, whether this was before or after the allocation of the clusters to the intervention groups, and whether the person recruiting the subject was blind to the treatment allocation. For fuller discussion see Puffer *et al.* (2003). Kerry *et al.* (2005b) give an example of steps taken to reduce recruitment bias in a health education trial in rural Ghana where whole villages were randomised to intervention groups.

BOX 12.8 INFORMATION

Cluster trials: a summary

- ◆ Cluster trials randomly allocate *groups* of individuals, such as general practices or families, to receive the same intervention

- ◆ Individuals in clusters are not independent; they are more similar to each other than to individuals in other clusters. This non-independence affects sample size calculations and statistical analysis

- ◆ The intraclass correlation coefficient measures the degree of correlation between individuals within clusters, and is used in sample size calculations

- ◆ Cluster trials tend to need more subjects than individually randomised trials.

- ◆ Cluster trials have a certain number of clusters and a number of individuals within the clusters. This two-level structure must be taken into account in the statistical analysis

- ◆ Ignoring clustering in sample size calculations leads to underpowered studies

- ◆ Ignoring clustering in analysis leads to P values that are too small and confidence intervals that are too narrow

- ◆ Reporting full details of the cluster trial design and analysis is essential for other researchers to be able to interpret the findings

BOX 12.9 INFORMATION

Extended CONSORT for cluster trials—a summary

CONSORT for cluster trials: summary of items additional to main CONSORT checklist

- ◆ Make clear in title and/or abstract that trial is clustered

- ◆ Report the reasons for choosing a cluster design

- ◆ Report how effects of clustering were used in the sample size calculations, including reporting the intraclass correlation coefficient that was used

- ◆ Report how clustering was allowed for in the analysis

- ◆ Give a flowchart of both clusters and individuals from recruitment to analysis

- ◆ Present baseline group data for clusters and for individuals

- ◆ Report the intraclass correlation coefficient for the primary outcome of the trial

For full details see Campbell *et al.* (2004) or the CONSORT website

12.5 Presenting trials with other designs

At the time of writing, CONSORT guidelines for trials of the following designs are in preparation:

non-inferiority, cross-over, factorial, multi-arm, and within-subject. The website will provide up-to-date information on this continuously developing field.

However, the CONSORT statement for two-group trials is an invaluable checklist and guide in the absence of specific guidelines.

Chapter summary

Presenting a randomised controlled trial

Follow CONSORT guidelines for reporting randomised controlled trials. In particular:

◆ Ensure that the study is clearly reported as a randomised controlled trial so that it is indexed as a trial for other users to find in electronic searches

◆ Show a flowchart from recruitment to analysis to account for all participants

◆ Describe sample size calculations in detail

◆ Describe the randomisation process and any blinding in detail

◆ Describe the statistical methods including any adjustment of P values for multiple testing and any variables adjusted for

◆ Distinguish between planned and unplanned analyses

◆ Report the primary outcome prominently, whether significant or not

◆ Report all secondary outcomes, whether significant or not

◆ For all outcomes, give an effect size, and whenever possible also give a measure of precision (95% CI)

◆ Do not assume that 'not statistically significant' means 'there is no difference'; look at the effect size and the width of the confidence interval

◆ Follow CONSORT cluster guidelines if the unit of randomisation is a cluster

◆ See CONSORT extension for other trial designs

References

Altman DG (1991). *Practical Statistics for Medical Research*. London: Chapman and Hall.

Altman DG, Bland JM (1994). Diagnostic tests. 3: Receiver operating characteristic plots. *BMJ*, **309**, 188.

Altman DG, Machin D, Bryant TN, Gardner MJ (eds) (2000). *Statistics with Confidence* (2nd edn) London: BMJ Books.

Altman DG, Schulz KF, Moher D, *et al.* (2001). The revised CONSORT statement for reporting randomized trials: explanation and elaboration. *Ann Intern Med*, **134**, 663–694.

Anderson HR, Ayres JG, Sturdy PM, *et al.* (2005). Bronchodilator treatment and deaths from asthma: case–control study. *BMJ*, **330**, 117–120.

Armitage P, Berry G, Matthews JNS (2002). *Statistical Methods in Medical Research* (4th edn) Oxford: Blackwell Science.

Barnes PM, Price L, Maddocks A, Lyons RA, Nash P, McCabe M (2001). Unnecessary school absence after minor injury: case–control study. *BMJ*, **323**, 1034–1035.

Begg C, Cho M, Eastwood S, *et al.* (1996). Improving the quality of reporting of randomized controlled trials. The CONSORT statement. *JAMA*, **276**, 637–639.

Bland M (2000). *An Introduction to Medical Statistics* (3rd edn) Oxford: Oxford University Press.

Bland M, Peacock J (2000). *Statistical Questions in Evidence-based Medicine*. Oxford: Oxford University Press.

Bolliger CT, Zellweger JP, Danielsson T, *et al.* (2000). Smoking reduction with oral nicotine inhalers: double blind, randomised clinical trial of efficacy and safety. *BMJ*, **321**, 329–333.

Brooke OG, Anderson HR, Bland JM, Peacock JL, Stewart CM (1989). Effects on birth weight of smoking, alcohol, caffeine, socioeconomic factors, and psychosocial stress. *BMJ*, **298**, 795–801.

Bruce M, Peacock JL, Iverson A, Wolfe C (2001). Hepatitis B and HIV antenatal screening. 2: User survey. *BJ Midwifery*, **9**, 640–645.

Campbell MJ, Machin D (1999). *Medical Statistics: A Commonsense Approach* (3rd edn). Chichester: Wiley.

Campbell MJ (2001). *Statistics at Square Two: Understanding Modern Statistical Applications in Medicine*. London: BMJ Books.

Campbell MK, Elbourne DR, Altman DG (2004). CONSORT statement: extension to cluster randomised trials. *BMJ*, **328**, 702–708.

Cappuccio FP, Cook DG, Atkinson RW, Strazzullo P (1997). Prevalence, detection, and management of cardiovascular risk factors in different ethnic groups in south London. *Heart*, **78**, 555–563.

Connor J, Norton R, Ameratunga S, *et al.* (2002). Driver sleepiness and risk of serious injury to car occupants: population based case control study. *BMJ*, **324**, 1125–1128.

Cook DG, Peacock JL, Feyerabend C, *et al.* (1996). Relation of caffeine intake and blood caffeine concentrations during pregnancy to fetal growth: prospective population based study. *BMJ*, **313**, 1358–1362.

Davies HT, Crombie IK, Tavakoli M (1998). When can odds ratios mislead? *BMJ*, **316**, 989–991.

Donner A, Klar N (2000). *Design and Analysis of Cluster Randomization Trials in Health Research*. London: Arnold.

Greenough A, Limb E, Marston L, Marlow N, Calvert S, Peacock J (2005). Risk factors for respiratory morbidity in infancy after very premature birth. *Arch Dis Child Fetal Neonatal Ed*, **90**, F320–F323.

Hawton K, Simkin S, Deeks JJ, *et al.* (1999). Effects of a drug overdose in a television drama on presentations to hospital for self poisoning: time series and questionnaire study. *BMJ*, **318**, 972–977.

Hoek G, Brunekreef B, Kosterink P, Van den Berg R, Hofschreuder P (1993). Effect of ambient ozone on peak expiratory flow of exercising children in The Netherlands. *Arch Environ Health*, **48**, 27–32.

Hollis S, Campbell F (1999). What is meant by intention to treat analysis? Survey of published randomised controlled trials. *BMJ*, **319**, 670–674.

Johnson AH, Peacock JL, Greenough A, *et al.* (2002). High-frequency oscillatory ventilation for the prevention of chronic lung disease of prematurity. *N Engl J Med*, 347, 633–642.

Johnson S, Marlow N, Wolke D, *et al.* (2004). Validation of a parent report measure of cognitive development in very preterm infants. *Dev Med Child Neurol*, 46, 389–397.

Kerry SM, Bland JM (1998a). Sample size in cluster randomisation. *BMJ*, **316**, 549.

Kerry SM, Bland JM (1998b). Analysis of a trial randomised in clusters. *BMJ*, **316**, 54.

Kerry S, Oakeshott P, Dundas D, Williams J (2000). Influence of postal distribution of the Royal College of Radiologists' guidelines, together with feedback on radiological referral rates, on X-ray referrals from general practice: a randomized controlled trial. *Fam Pract*, 17, 46–52.

Kerry SM, Micah FB, Plange-Rhule J, Eastwood JB, Cappuccio FP (2005a). Blood pressure and body mass index in lean rural and semi-urban subjects in West Africa. *J Hypertens*, 23, 1645–1651.

Kerry SM, Cappuccio FP, Emmett L, Plange-Rhule J, Eastwood JB (2005b). Reducing selection bias in a cluster randomized trial in West African villages. *Clin Trials*, 2, 125–129.

Kirkwood BR, Sterne JAC (2003). *Essential Medical Statistics* (2nd edn). Oxford: Blackwell Science.

Machin D, Campbell MJ, Fayers PM, Pinol A (1997). *Sample Size Tables for Clinical Studies* (2nd edn). Oxford: Blackwell Science.

Meyer LC, Peacock JL, Bland JM, Anderson HR (1994). Symptoms and health problems in pregnancy: their association with social factors, smoking, alcohol, caffeine and attitude to pregnancy. *Paediatr Perinat Epidemiol* 8, 145–155.

Miller MA, Kerry SM, Cook DG, Cappuccio FP (2004). Cellular adhesion molecules and blood pressure: interaction with sex in a multi ethnic population. *J Hypertens* 22, 705–11.

Missouris CG, Kalaitzidis RG, Kerry SM, Cappuccio FP (2004). Predictors of mortality on patients with peripheral vascular disease: a prospective follow-up study. *BJ Diabetes Vasc Dis*, 4, 196–200.

Moher D, Schulz KF, Altman DG (2001). The CONSORT statement: revised recommendations for improving the quality of reports of parallel-group randomised trials. *Lancet*, 357, 1191–1194.

Nam JM, Blackwelder WC (2002). Analysis of the ratio of marginal probabilities in a matched-pair setting. *Stat Med*, 21, 689–699.

Oakeshott P, Kerry S, Hay S, Hay P (1998). Opportunistic screening for chlamydial infection at time of cervical smear testing in general practice: prevalence study. *BMJ*, 316, 351–352.

Oakeshott P, Hay P, Hay S, *et al.* (2002). Detection of Chlamydia trachomatis infection in early pregnancy using self-administered vaginal swabs and first pass urines: a cross-sectional community-based survey. *Br J Gen Pract*, 52, 830–832.

Oakeshott P, Kerry S, Dean S, Cappuccio F (2005). Nurse-led management of hypertension. *Br J Gen Pract*, 55, 53–54.

Parmar MKB, Machin D (1995). *Survival Analysis: A Practical Approach*. Chichester: Wiley.

Peacock JL, Bland JM, Anderson HR (1991). Effects on birthweight of alcohol and caffeine consumption in smoking women. *J Epidemiol Community Health*, 45, 159–163.

Peacock JL, Cook DG, Carey IM, *et al.* (1998). Maternal cotinine level during pregnancy and birthweight for gestational age. *Int J Epidemiol*, 27, 647–656.

Peacock JL, Symonds P, Jackson P, *et al.* (2003). Acute effects of winter air pollution on respiratory function in schoolchildren in southern England. *Occup Environ Med*, 60, 82–89.

Peacock PJ, Peacock JL, Victor CR, Chazot C (2005). Changes in the emergency workload of the London Ambulance Service between 1989 and 1999. *Emerg Med J*, 22, 56–59.

Peduzzi P, Concato J, Feinstein AR, Holford TR (1995). Importance of events per independent variable in proportional hazards regression analysis. II. Accuracy and precision of regression estimates. *J Clin Epidemiol*, 48, 1503–1510.

Peduzzi P, Concato J, Kemper E, Holford TR, Feinstein AR (1996). A simulation study of the number of events per variable in logistic regression analysis. *J Clin Epidemiol*, 49, 1373–1379.

Petrie A, Sabin C (2000). *Medical Statistics at a Glance*. Oxford: Blackwell Science.

Pocock SJ, Clayton TC, Altman DG (2002). Survival plots of time-to-event outcomes in clinical trials: good practice and pitfalls. *Lancet*, 359, 1686–1689.

Puffer S, Torgerson D, Watson J (2003). Evidence for risk of bias in cluster randomised trials: review of recent trials published in three general medical journals. *BMJ*, 327, 785–789.

Schrader H, Stovner LJ, Helde G, Sand T, Bovim G (2001). Prophylactic treatment of migraine with angiotensin converting enzyme inhibitor (lisinopril): randomised, placebo controlled, crossover study. *BMJ*, 322, 19–22.

Spence DP, Hotchkiss J, Williams CS, Davies PD (1993). Tuberculosis and poverty. *BMJ*, 307, 759–761.

Steptoe A, Perkins-Porras L, McKay C, Rink E, Hilton S, Cappuccio FP (2003). Behavioural counselling to increase consumption of fruit and vegetables in low income adults: randomised trial. *BMJ*, 326, 855–858.

Stewart G, Ruggles R, Peacock J (2004). The association of self-reported violence at home and health in primary school pupils in West London. *J Public Health (Oxf)*, 26, 19–23.

Swinscow TDV, Campbell MJ (2002). *Statistics at Square One*. (10th edn). London: BMJ Books.

Thomas MR, Rafferty GF, Limb ES, *et al.* (2004). Pulmonary function at follow-up of very preterm infants from the United Kingdom oscillation study. *Am J Respir Crit Care Med*, 169, 868–872.

Thompson SG, Barber JA (2000). How should cost data in pragmatic randomised trials be analysed? *BMJ*, 320, 1197–1200.

UK BEAM Trial Team (2004). United Kingdom back pain exercise and manipulation (UK BEAM) randomised trial: effectiveness of physical treatments for back pain in primary care. *BMJ*, **329**, 1377–1381.

Whincup PH, Gilg JA, Emberson JR, *et al.* (2004). Passive smoking and risk of coronary heart disease and stroke: prospective study with cotinine measurement. *BMJ*, **329**, 200–205.

Yu CK, Papageorghiou AT, Boli A, Cacho AM, Nicolaides KH (2002). Screening for pre-eclampsia and fetal growth restriction in twin pregnancies at 23 weeks of gestation by transvaginal uterine artery Doppler. *Ultrasound Obstet Gynecol*, **20**, 535–540.

Web references

http://www.brunel.ac.uk/about/acad/health/healthstaff/profiles/stafflistmtor/peacock/peacockpublications/
http://www.cardiff.ac.uk/medicine/epidemiology_statistics/research/statistics/proportions.htm
http://www.cdc.gov/epiinfo/
http://www.consort-statement.org
http://www.corec.org.uk/
http://www.dh.gov.uk/PublicationsAndStatistics/Publications/PublicationsPolicyAndGuidance/
   PublicationsPolicyAndGuidanceArticle/fs/en?CONTENT_ID=4005727&chk=CNcpyR
http://www.formrecognition.com/
http://www.sgul.ac.uk/depts/phs/guide/methods.htm
http://www.som.soton.ac.uk/cia/main.htm
http://www.stata.com/stb/stb59
http://www.statsdirect.com/
http://www.statsolusa.com
http://www-users.york.ac.uk/~mb55/soft/soft.htm

Index to boxes and figures